LEARNING EVIDENCE-BASED RESEARCH SKILLS THE PEAK PRACTICE WAY

A Beginner's Guide

LEARNING EVIDENCE-BASED RESEARCH SKILLS THE PEAK PRACTICE WAY

A Beginner's Guide

DEBRA R. HANNA

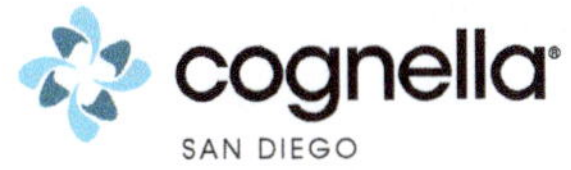

SAN DIEGO

Bassim Hamadeh, CEO and Publisher
Amanda Martin, Publisher
Amy Smith, Senior Project Editor
Alia Bales, Production Manager
Emely Villavicencio, Senior Graphic Designer
Kylie Bartolome, Licensing Specialist
Natalie Piccotti, Director of Marketing
Kassie Graves, Senior Vice President, Editorial

Printed in the United States of America.

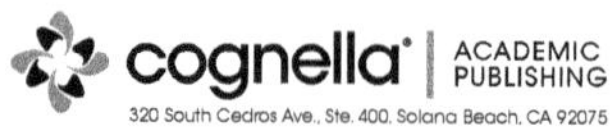

ACTIVE LEARNING

This book has interactive activities available to complement your reading.

Your instructor may have customized the selection of activities available for your unique course. Please check with your professor to verify whether your class will access this content through the Cognella Active Learning portal (http://active.cognella.com) or through your home learning management system.

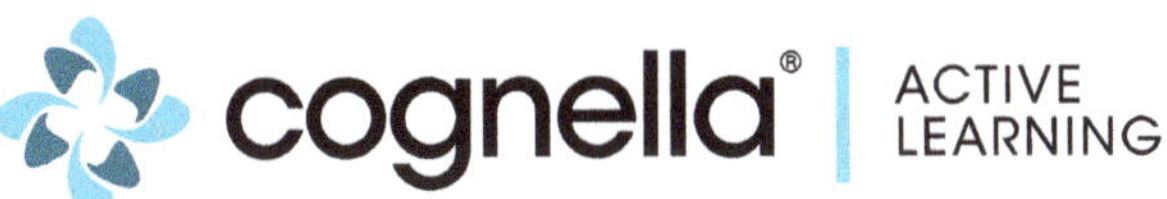

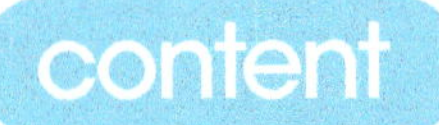

Brief Contents

Detailed Contents

PART II Building Evidence-Based Research Skills 45

Preface

The idea for this three-book series about evidence-based research skills came to me several years ago when I struggled to find the right book to teach a graduate-level course. I felt a bit like the professor's version of Goldilocks. Instead of finding bowls of porridge or chairs or beds that were too large, too small, too hard, too soft, I found textbooks that were too simple, too complex, too costly, too confusing. It was a labor of love to find an affordable, well-written textbook that was just right. Graduate students need more depth and breadth than undergrad students but less than doctoral students.

In March 2019 I spoke at the Case Western Reserve University nursing theory conference. At the heart of my speech, later published as an article, was the "simple idea about four learner levels and the corresponding kinds of nursing practice related to each level of education" (Hanna, 2019, 2020). That morning I linked each learner level (Undergraduate, Graduate, Doctor of Nursing Practice, and Research Doctorate) with relevant teaching strategies and standards. I quoted the French Dominican theologian Fr. Sertillanges, O. P. (1946/1987), who wrote: "The wise man [sic] begins at the beginning and does not take a second step until he is sure of the first." Fr. Sertillanges's idea was that every professional person starts their formal education at the most basic level. In time, as they gain experience and higher levels of education, some professionals develop deep intellectual lives. Society benefits from the fruitfulness of professional people's intellectual lives.

My claim that morning was that nursing, like most practice professions, is not a Do-It-Yourself endeavor. Rather, I proposed that nurse scholars might consider writing "a series of progressive nursing knowledge textbooks" at several learner levels. If so, undergrad students' textbooks would be written at a level appropriate for novices with no knowledge or experience in nursing. Graduate students' books would be written for nurses with experience and an undergraduate education. Doctoral students' books would be at higher, more complex levels needed for evidence-based research translation (DNP) or for primary research productivity (PhD).

This three-book series about evidence-based research skills fulfills what I proposed that day. Each book is written for one of three distinct learner levels. The first book, *Learning Evidence-Based Research Skills the Peak Practice Way: A Beginner's Guide*, is for readers who have no prior knowledge of research or evidence-based practice. The focus of the beginner's guide is on the language and research context of nine basic skills. Intended readers for the beginner's guide include undergraduate students and possibly high school advanced practice students who are eligible to take college courses.

The second book, *Advancing Evidence-Based Research Skills the Peak Practice Way*, is written for graduate students with experience in their field who have some grasp of research, but who have not yet had much chance to conduct research. This second book goes into greater depth about research methods, threats to validity, statistical analysis, narrative analysis, and a few more evidence-based research skills.

The third book, *Achieving Evidence-Based Research Expertise the Peak Practice Way*, is like the "Top Gun" approach to learning. The third book will be valuable for students engaged in doctoral studies, as well as anyone who teaches evidence-based research skills to others. This book is written to challenge in-depth knowledge with samples of ambiguous research choices. Its purpose is to help experienced evidence-based researchers hone their expertise to solve complex problems.

Some readers might wonder what "the peak practice way" is. Peak practice is not my idea. It was the lifelong work of the late Dr. K. Anders Ericsson (1947–2020). I was introduced to Dr. Ericsson's work when I read about the 10,000 hours rule in Malcolm Gladwell's 2008 *New York Times* bestseller *Outliers: The Story of Success*. Gladwell's account of how the Beatles became the Beatles inspired me to search for and start using Dr. Ericsson's scholarly work in my own teaching. Ericsson's 2016 book, coauthored with Robert Pool, was called *PEAK: Secrets from the New Science of Expertise.* I have written this book series using Dr. Ericsson's peak practice principles of purposeful practice, adaptability, mental representations, and deliberate practice, with the hope that as his ideas live on in these books, they will help readers achieve true evidence-based research expertise.

Debra R. Hanna, New York City, April 13, 2023

References

Andersson, E., & Pool, R. (2016). *Peak: Secrets from the New Science of Expertise.* Mariner Books.

Gladwell, M. (2008). *Outliers: The Story of Success.* Little, Brown, and Company.

Hanna, D. R. (March 24, 2019). *Differentiated Standards for Teaching at Four Learner Levels* [Podium presentation]. Nursing Theory Conference, Cleveland, OH, United States.

Hanna, D. R. (2020). Proposing Standards for Teaching Authentic Nursing Knowledge. *Advances in Nursing Science, 43*(1), 42–49.

Sertillanges, A. G. (1987). *The Intellectual Life: Its Spirit, Conditions, Methods* (M. Ryan, Trans.). Catholic University of America (Original work published 1946).

List of Reviewers

Sharon E. Bigger, PhD, MA, RN, CHPN, CNE
East Tennessee State University

Angeline Bushy, PhD, RN, FAAN
Professor, Bert Fish Eminent Chair
University of Central Florida, College of Nursing

Susan Davidson, EdD, APRN, NP-C
Professor and Coordinator, RN-BSN Gateway Program
The University of Tennessee at Chattanooga (UTC), School of Nursing

Melissa B. Miner DNP, RN, CNE
Pennsylvania State University

Kathryn Niemeyer PhD, MSc, MSN, FNP-BC
Ferris State University, School of Nursing

Somer Nourse DNP, RN, CNE
Associate Professor of Nursing
Indiana State University, School of Nursing

Jill Parsons PhD, RN, CNE
McKendree University

Catherine A. Schmitt PhD RN
University of Wisconsin Oshkosh, College of Nursing

Ernest Smith
Northern Kentucky University

Jane A. Tiedt, PhD, RN, ANEF
Professor of Nursing
Gonzaga University, School of Nursing & Human Physiology

Introduction

This first book in the series on evidence-based research skills is for beginners. It is for readers who have never learned about scientific research or evidence-based practice. This book includes content to build the language and context that readers need for evidence-based research. Readers will learn and practice nine basic skills. The intended audience is undergraduate college students, high school advanced placement students, or any professional person who wants to learn evidence-based research skills.

Readers might wonder why this book refers to evidence-based research skills instead of evidence-based practice (EBP). Excellent textbooks that address the full scope of evidence-based practice exist. This author believes that evidence-based practice is a complete program of activities and skills. EBP supports a collaborative, team-based approach to clinical and professional decision making. This book provides a practical view of evidence-based research. It teaches nine essential evidence-based research skills that all evidence-based researchers need. The evidence-based research skills described in this book are a subset of the full scope of evidence-based practice skills.

How to Use This Book

This book is set up with practice exercises. Readers who have never conducted an evidence-based research project will be able to set up, conduct, complete, and report a simple project to their peers and others. By using the tables and practice exercises provided, readers should succeed. A PowerPoint template shows how evidence-based research projects flow.

The Language of Evidence-Based Research

Learning the language of evidence-based research starts with pre-chapter language guides before chapters 1–4 which can be accessed in Active Learning. The language guide, called Another Name For, defines words introduced for the first time. The Also Known As guide shows "close cousin" words, which are other words for the same idea. Using the language guides will help readers smoothly grasp each chapter's content. Ideas defined in pre-chapter language guides give readers context to understand the chapter's content.

For example, beginners can have trouble seeing the difference between research studies, called "non-experimental," and scholarly articles, called "non-research." The two words, "non-experimental" and "non-research," sound alike. Before each chapter begins, language guides give definitions and close cousin examples to make language clear. "Non-experimental" refers to research that is descriptive in nature, where there is no experimental intervention. "Non-research" refers to articles that give an expert opinion. An expert opinion might use ideas from research, but the article itself is not a research report.

Process

Readers will profit from reading the complete book once through before starting a project. By reading the complete book readers will learn the language and ideas of scientific and evidence-based research. They will grasp the full evidence-based research process before starting a first project.

To conduct evidence-based research well, beginners must recognize ideas about scientific research, scholarly articles, search engines, and more. Section I, Chapters 1–4, provides basic understanding about these ideas.

Section II covers nine evidence-based research skills. To learn these skills well, it is best to work in an orderly way. This beginner's guide teaches skills one at a time. Books two and three of this series build proficiency and expertise, respectively.

The format for the entire three-book series is based on lifelong research by the late Dr. K. Anders Ericsson (1947–2020). Dr. Ericsson studied how people become experts (Ericsson & Pool, 2016). Each chapter includes separate peak practice exercises. Purposeful practice exercises are the easiest level of skill and knowledge acquisition. Purposeful practice includes practice to build memories. The language guides are at the level of purposeful practice. Section II exercises build on memories from the language guides in Section I.

Another type of peak practice exercise develops "mental representations." These exercises help readers learn with images and metaphors. A PowerPoint template and other images embedded in the book will help readers form mental representations. The last key to peak practice is to engage in deliberate practice exercises. Chances for deliberate practice skills are given in each skills chapter of this book.

Chapters start with a set of reader's learning goals. For nursing students, learning goals include the first level of learning outcomes from the American Association of Colleges of Nursing Essentials document from 2021. First-level outcomes are for prelicensure and undergraduate education, which is compatible with this book's audience. My hope is that by using all three books well, readers will grow from beginners to experts.

Are You Ready?

Undergraduate students typically learn how to read research reports. In contrast, graduate students learn how to conduct simple research studies. People pursuing research doctorates conduct substantial doctoral dissertation research studies to obtain degrees in basic, social, or human science disciplines.

In today's world, however, the need to translate primary scientific research into daily work practices has led academics from separate professional practice disciplines to create a second path to a terminal degree. The traditional research doctorate is no longer the only terminal degree. Three examples of practice-based terminal degrees are the DNP (Doctor of Nursing Practice), PharmD (Doctor of Pharmacology), and PsyD (Doctor of Clinical Psychology). Students who seek practice-based terminal degrees will benefit from additional content in books two and three. However, students at any level of education who lack a firm grasp of research or evidence-based practice knowledge might find this book helpful.

If this first book reads like an interesting story, with examples of an evidence-based research project in progress, readers will learn the language and skills to work independently.

Leaders in industries such as healthcare, education, and business expect professional people to conduct evidence-based research projects. The idea is that evidence-based research improves work quality and efficiency. Readers who need these skills but who have not yet had the necessary education have the right book in hand. May you enjoy this reading journey!

PART I

A Practical View of Evidence-Based Research

CHAPTER 1

Tell an Evidence Story

LEARNING GOALS

1. Explain what an evidence story is.
2. Describe stakeholder roles.
3. Use the PowerPoint template to explain the logical flow of evidence-based research.

The Evidence Story

In *The Poetics*, Aristotle said that all stories have three basic parts: a beginning, a middle, and an end. Aristotle also said that good stories are logical. This chapter uses a PowerPoint template to show the logic of an evidence story from beginning to end.

What is an **evidence story**? An evidence story is the full account of an evidence-based research project from start to finish. The full account is presented to others once the evidence-based research project ends. The evidence story starts with a question about two separate ways to reach an outcome. Once the question is clear, researchers use a formal process to seek relevant evidence. Researchers use inclusion and exclusion criteria to screen potential evidence. After the initial screening process, researchers decide on a final set of articles, the evidence set. Then researchers use critical appraisal skills to evaluate the evidence. During critical appraisal, researchers transfer data to a variety of evidence tables. The evidence tables display key findings about interventions, comparison interventions, and outcomes. After researchers analyze the data, they synthesize it and create an evidence synthesis table. Synthesis builds the evidence story's ending, which answers the original question. Researchers present a logical evidence story with synthesized findings to other people, called stakeholders. Based on the evidence story, researchers might advise changes to work practices, if needed.

To recap Aristotle's idea, an evidence story starts at the beginning with a researcher's unanswered question. The middle of the evidence story is the most complex section, with two parts. Part 1 of the middle is the path to find evidence, also called the search strategy. Part 2 of the middle is the evidence analysis and synthesis. When it is complete, part 3 of the the evidence story shows how synthesized evidence credibly answers the question.

Evidence-based research is logical. Yet it takes time for beginners to learn the process. In this chapter, a generic PowerPoint template shows how to build a complete, logical evidence story. Readers will see how an evidence story evolves. The template shows readers nine basic skills needed to conduct a simple evidence-based research project. Readers who want to develop their expertise further will benefit from reading books two and three.

Telling the Evidence Story to Stakeholders

Another aspect of an evidence-based research project is to tell the evidence story to all relevant **stakeholders**. Two groups of potential stakeholders exist. The first group is people who must know about the project before it begins. Work supervisors might need to approve the researcher's use of work time for a project. The first presentation, before any research starts, could be to the researcher's direct supervisor. If researchers collaborate with a team of professional peers, one presentation might be to coworkers. In certain work settings, research teams might need additional approval from committees. Anyone who approves an evidence-based research project before it begins is a stakeholder.

After a project ends, researchers will present their findings to the same stakeholders who approved the project. However, researchers might also present to other stakeholders. Those stakeholders are people who want to know the answer after the evidence-based research project ends. Anyone directly affected by a project's outcomes is a stakeholder. For example, if an evidence-based research project leads to changes in work procedures or policies, workers affected by those changes will want to hear the evidence story. If researchers advise changes to standards, policies, or procedures, additional stakeholders might be committee members who oversee standards, policies, or procedures. Stakeholders are people who have a "stake" in the topic. They will want to hear the complete evidence story.

Researchers who conduct evidence-based research projects independently (without a work team and not during one's work hours) would not notify work supervisors. Yet, when an independent project ends, evidence-based researchers might share their findings and advice with stakeholders beyond their work setting.

An Evidence Story PowerPoint Template

The PowerPoint template has 30 slides. Selected slides below show how an evidence-based research project can unfold. The slide numbers given below match with the template.

Slide 1: Title Slide

CONCISE WORKING TITLE
(*put a "working" title here*)
Your name, title
Your institution
Date of Presentation, Venue
Your contact information

IMG 1.1

Most projects and presentations start with a concise working title. For example, a study has a full title of "Helping Teenage Parents of Premature Babies Avoid Hospital Readmissions." The concise working title might be "Teen Parents of Neonates." During a project, it is best to use a concise working title. When researchers finish their work, they often have new insights about their topic through the evidence they have analyzed. Those insights affect how researchers might reword their project's final title.

Slide 4: Background and Significance Slide

The background slide provides context and rationale for the evidence-based research. Give background information in one or two bullets. Researchers explain why this research question arose.

The project's significance is the importance of an evidence-based research project. Significance has various dimensions. How frequently a problem occurs can be what makes a problem important to study. How large, serious, or severe the problem is might make it important to study. The human or economic costs linked with that problem can be sizable. Unmet desired outcomes or failure to prevent undesired outcomes can be good reasons to study a problem. These examples are all types of significance. To tell an evidence story, the background and significance slides create context for the evidence-based research question.

Slide 6: Foreground (Or P-I-C-O) Question

The Foreground Question

The foreground question was:

Chapter 5 has information about P-I-C-O questions.

Evidence-based research projects are built to answer foreground questions

IMG 1.2

Evidence-based research requires specially worded questions, called the **P-I-C-O** or **foreground questions.** Chapter 5 has more information about P-I-C-O questions. Evidence-based researchers write foreground questions with a PICO or PICOT format. P-I-C-O is an acronym, pronounced "pee-ko." The letters stand for **P**opulation, **I**ntervention, **C**omparison Intervention, and **O**utcome. Sometimes, there is a fifth letter, T, which stands for **T**ime Frame to achieve the outcome.

Slide 7: Elements of the PICO/T Question

PICO/T QUESTION (STATE THE PICO/T QUESTION; WRITE EACH ELEMENT OF THE QUESTION. THE ELEMENTS MIGHT BE REFINED LATER ON)

P= Population/Patients

I= Intervention

C= Comparison

O= Outcome

T= Time to achieve the outcome

In ______(P), how does ______(I) compared with______(C) affect _____(O) within ______(T)?

IMG 1.3

Researchers write precise PICO questions first by naming each element. The PICO question elements help researchers set up a search strategy to seek evidence from library databases. The PICO elements are (**P**) for **P**opulation X, (**I**) for **I**ntervention A, (**C**) for **C**omparison Intervention B, and (**O**) for **O**utcome Y. Notice the relationship between P and O. When the Population word is linked in the question to the Outcome word, this is the "right" relationship between P and O. The P and O words are the subject and object of the sentence. Keep in mind that an object fulfills the subject's action. Chapter 5 has more detailed content.

Likewise, notice the relationship between the I word and the C word. When the intervention word links to the comparison intervention word, they are in "right" relationship. The comparison of two interventions (or two ways to achieve an outcome) strengthens an evidence-based question. The two interventions are the action words in the question. A common evidence-based question format is: For population X (the P element), how does Intervention A (the I element) compared with Comparison Intervention B (the C element) affect Outcome Y (the O element)? Chapter 5, "Pose Precise PICO Questions," explains this first skill in detail. A separate PP template slide shows the final PICO question in proper format.

Slide 9: The PICO Question

PICO QUESTION

Put your final PICO question here in proper format

IM3 1.4

Building a Resilient Search Strategy

The next stage of evidence-based research is to conduct a formal search for published evidence in library databases. This area is where experienced investigators work in overlapping, interrelated ways on multiple project aspects at one time. Besides building a resilient search strategy, investigators must keep track of their search efforts and results. When researchers tell the evidence story, each step must be clear to stakeholders. When investigators complete their evidence-based project, researchers have a duty to report their search path and findings to stakeholders in an explicit way. Use a search figure like the one in Slide 11 to show the stages of the search and all its elements. Stages of the search are listed on the left side: identification, screening, eligibility, and included. Transparency is the key for stakeholders to see the research as credible.

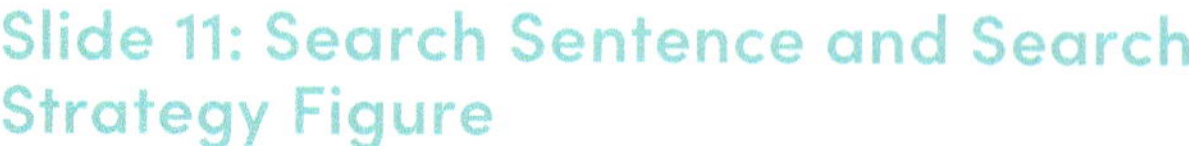

Slide 11: Search Sentence and Search Strategy Figure

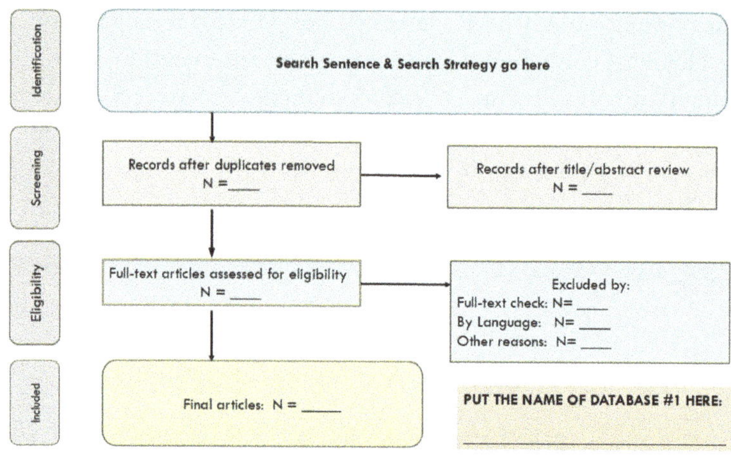

IMG 1.5

When researchers are transparent about their search strategy, they help others replicate their efforts from the Search Figure. People can judge whether the evidence is valid, reliable, and credible. Stakeholders will see if advice is **evidence-based**. Reporting unclear paths to evidence can lead stakeholders to suspect the findings. People reject advice perceived as biased, incomplete, or trivial. More about the ethics of evidence-based versus evidence-*biased* research is in Chapter 4.

Select Library Databases

Healthcare professionals, such as physicians, nurses, social workers, and therapists for art, music, communication & speech, physical, and occupational therapy will be more likely to use PubMed, Medline, or CINAHL for their searches. However, additional databases are available, such as Psychlit, ERIC, and Web of Science. Databases are different from each other in terms of the number of journals each database holds and how the databases operate. Each database has its own search rules. Chapters 7 and 8 discuss searches in detail.

TABLE 1.1 Table to Record Search Decisions

DATABASE name						
PICO words: starter search terms	Date/ Time of the search	Close cousin words	Filters/ Limits	Boolean Operators	# Hits	Decision

Build Strong Search Strategies

Investigators must build good search strategies to search at least two databases. Before building the search strategy, it is important for investigators to be familiar with the database's search rules. Chapter 7 presents database search rules in detail. It is important for all investigators to keep track of all the information and data for each search (see Table 1.1).

There is a difference between PICO search terms, Filters, Limits, and Boolean Operators. Textbooks often refer to synonyms. In this beginner's guide, the phrase "close cousin words" replaces the word "synonyms" for specific reasons. Chapter 6 and Chapter 7 explain search strategy ideas in detail.

Inclusion and Exclusion Criteria

Slide 13: Inclusion and Exclusion Criteria

INCLUSION AND EXCLUSION CRITERIA [ON THIS SLIDE YOU'LL PUT THE INCLUSION/EXCLUSION CRITERIA FOR YOUR KEEPER ARTICLES; CAN FILL THIS IN BEFORE YOUR SEARCH AND WILL REFINE IT LATER]

Inclusion criteria

Which articles would be included?

Exclusion criteria

Which articles would be excluded?

IMG 1.6

The original meaning for the phrase "**inclusion and exclusion criteria**" was to guide eligibility of human volunteers for research studies. "Inclusion criteria" are all the traits that volunteers must have to be eligible for a study. "Exclusion criteria" are all the factors that might still exclude otherwise eligible volunteers. For example, a researcher wants to study daily activity levels of pregnant females during the second trimester of pregnancy. Exclusion criteria would be females who are not pregnant, or whose pregnancies are less than 13 weeks or more than 27 weeks. Another important exclusion criterion would be females in their second trimester who are confined to bed or are paralyzed and unable to move voluntarily.

In contrast with human subjects, samples for evidence-based research use published articles, not human volunteers. Novice researchers often misunderstand the role that inclusion and exclusion criteria play in a search for evidence. Inclusion criteria are the ideas that articles must have in order to be useful as evidence. Exclusion criteria mean the ideas or traits that articles must not have. Inclusion and exclusion criteria are not opposites. Evidence-based researchers who approach their search strategy with poorly considered criteria often have a superficial or incomplete search. Researchers must know which factors will exclude articles and which factors are needed before articles can be included in the final set of evidence.

As the search strategy unfolds, investigators use database tools, such as filters and limits, in analytical ways to create the search strategy. Two things are important for a good search strategy. First, exclude articles that can overwhelm the search. Second, include relevant published articles with information to answer the research question.

Slide 15: Types of Evidence Table

TYPES OF EVIDENCE TABLE

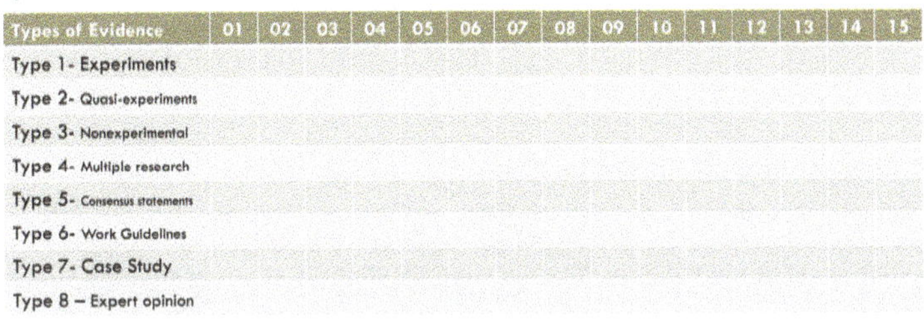

Types of Evidence	01	02	03	04	05	06	07	08	09	10	11	12	13	14	15
Type 1- Experiments															
Type 2- Quasi-experiments															
Type 3- Nonexperimental															
Type 4- Multiple research															
Type 5- Consensus statements															
Type 6- Work Guidelines															
Type 7- Case Study															
Type 8 – Expert opinion															

KEY: 01 Author, year; 02 Author xxxx; 03 Author xxxx; 04 Author xxxx; 05 Author xxxx; 06 Author xxxx; 07 Author xxxx; 08 Author xxxx; 09 Author xxxx; 10 Author xxxx; 11 Author xxxx; 12 Author xxxx; 13 Author xxxx; 14 Author xxxx; 15 Author xxxx

IMG 1.7

The Types of Evidence table in this book uses a novel approach to categorize evidence. Evidence-based textbooks often use a pyramid to sort evidence into five, seven, or eight levels (Dang et al 2021; Melynyk and Fineout-Overholt 2023; Pollit and Beck 2017). This book uses two rectangular figures, one for research and the other for non-research. Each figure has four types of evidence. This author believes rectangular figures will help novices learn about types of evidence. Chapter 8 has more details.

Slide 17: Critical Appraisal—Individual Article

CRITICAL APPRAISAL– INDIVIDUAL ARTICLE

01	Author names. (year). Article title. *Journal title, vol.# (issue #): page numbers*				
Category & Type of evidence: Research 1,2,3,4 **Nonresearch** 5,6,7,8	**Method** **Quant** Experimental Quasi-experimental Nonexperimental **Qual** Phenomenology Grounded Theory Ethnography **Mixed Methods**	**Sample** Population Sample size N=___ Type of sample	**Variables** Concepts Interventions (IV) Outcomes (DV) Themes	**Data collection** **Analysis** **Instruments**	**Findings** **Strengths** **Limits** **Interpretation**
Author credentials		**Reviewer's comments:**			**Quality of evidence**

IMG 1.8

Careful critical appraisal of evidence is a key to the quality of evidence-based research. Two tables show how to organize critical appraisal data gathered from the evidence. Chapter 10 has in-depth information about this skill.

Slide 18: Critical Appraisal Summary Table

Critical Appraisal Summary Table

Article #	Author	Pub Year	Study Category	Study Method	Sample Type	Sample Size	Ind Variable or topic	Dep variable	Measures Data Analysis	Findings	Type & Quality
01											
02											
03											
04											
05											
06											
07											
08											

KEY; 01 Author, XXXX; 02 Author XXXX; 03 Author XXXX; 04 Author XXXX; 05 Author XXXX; 06 Author XXXX; 07 Author XXXX; 08 Author XXXX;

IMG 1.9

Slide 19: Evidence Display Table: Interventions

EVIDENCE TABLE: INTERVENTION VARIABLES

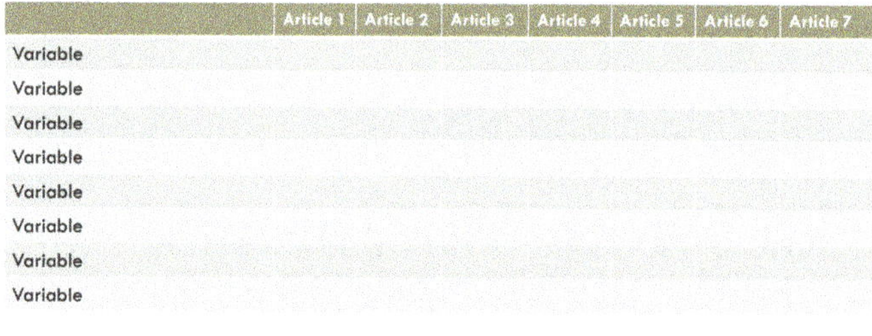

	Article 1	Article 2	Article 3	Article 4	Article 5	Article 6	Article 7
Variable							
Variable							
Variable							
Variable							
Variable							
Variable							
Variable							
Variable							

KEY; 01 Author, XXXX; 02 Author XXXX; 03 Author XXXX; 04 Author XXXX; 05 Author XXXX; 06 Author XXXX; 07 Author XXXX

IMG 1.10

Evidence display tables show where the evidence is present. The Social Determinants of Health table displays missing evidence. Evidence display tables can have a variety of elements represented. Researchers might need three or more tables per category to display all the data.

Slide 20: Evidence Display Table: SDOH Variables

EVIDENCE TABLE: SDOH VARIABLES

	Article 1	Article 2	Article 3	Article 4	Article 5	Article 6	Article 7
Variable							
Variable							
Variable							
Variable							
Variable							
Variable							
Variable							
Variable							

KEY; 01 Author, XXXX; 02 Author XXXX; 03 Author XXXX; 04 Author XXXX; 05 Author XXXX; 06 Author XXXX; 07 Author XXXX

IMG 1.11

Slide 21: Evidence Display Table: Outcomes

EVIDENCE TABLE: OUTCOMES VARIABLES

	Article 1	Article 2	Article 3	Article 4	Article 5	Article 6	Article 7
Variable							
Variable							
Variable							
Variable							
Variable							
Variable							
Variable							
Variable							

KEY; 01 Author, XXXX; 02 Author XXXX; 03 Author XXXX; 04 Author XXXX; 05 Author XXXX; 06 Author XXXX; 07 Author XXXX

IMG 1.12

Slide 22: Evidence Table: Synthesis

SYNTHESIS TABLE: TELL THE EVIDENCE STORY

	Article 1	Article 2	Article 3	Article 4	Article 5	Article 6	Article 7
Variable							
Variable							
Variable							
Variable							
Variable							
Variable							
Variable							
Variable							

KEY; 01 Author, XXXX; 02 Author XXXX; 03 Author XXXX; 04 Author XXXX; 05 Author XXXX; 06 Author XXXX; 07 Author XXXX

IMG 1.13

After displaying the evidence in tables, researchers synthesize the evidence and display it with icons that will "tell the evidence story." This table will show positive and negative outcomes, or increased or decreased outcomes. This table is where the original question is finally "answered."

Slide 23: Interpretation of Evidence

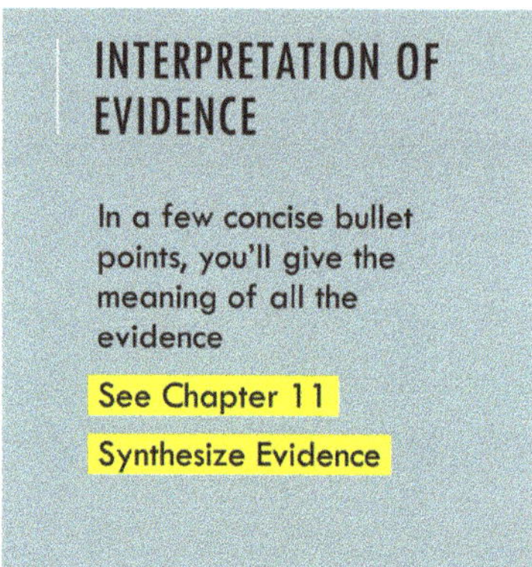

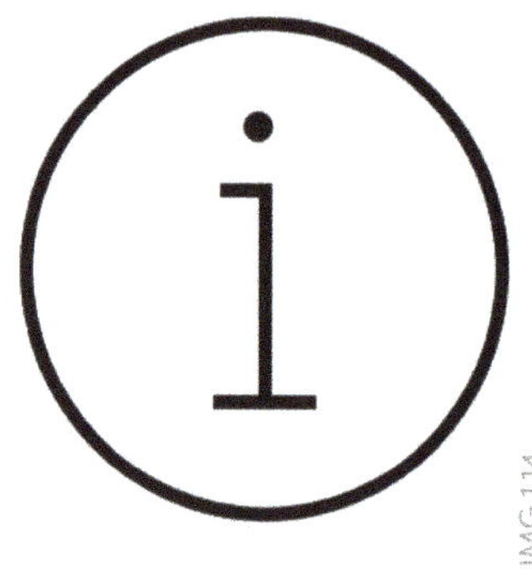

IMG 1.14

Interpretation of evidence follows synthesis, because interpretation gives valuable meaning to the synthesis of all the evidence shown in the previous slide.

Slide 24: Themes or Patterns of Evidence

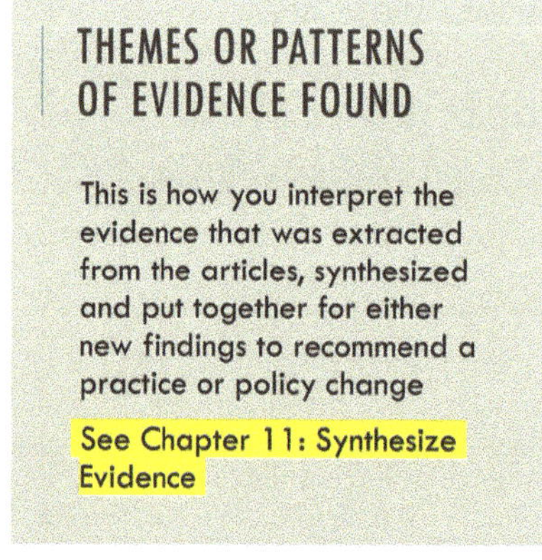

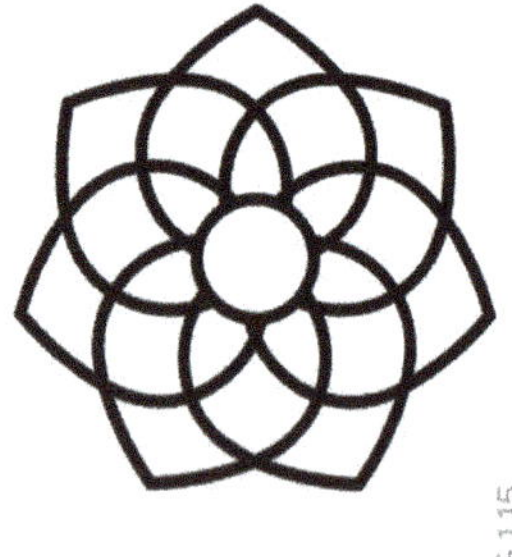

IMG 1.15

Research evidence can show important themes or patterns to answer the PICO question.

Slide 25: Implications of the Findings

CURRENT IMPLICATIONS OF THE FINDINGS

Clinical Implications	Actions to be taken
Clinical Practice – Generalist	xxxx
Clinical Practice – Advanced practice	xxxx
Organizational Policies/procedures	xxxx
Patient/Client education	xxxx
Improved Patient/Client Outcomes	xxxx
Patient/Client satisfaction: HCAHPS	xxxx
Nurse/Worker education	xxxx
Expenses: Costs to implement	xxxx
Revenue generated	xxxx
Revenue Reclaimed (Money saved)	xxxx

IMG 1.16

Researchers must state the evidence-based implications in three categories: current, future, and social determinants of health. Chapter 11 addresses this content.

Slide 28: Evidence-Based Advice and Advocacy

EVIDENCE-BASED ADVICE & ADVOCACY

Possible Categories of achievable actions advice

- Change work process, practices, or procedures
- Change policies, written procedures, or standards
- Change work flow between departments
- Advocate for change beyond the institution

IMG 1.17

As the evidence story ends, researchers give evidence-based advice for change (if needed) or affirm that the current intervention is sufficient.

Slide 29: Communication Plan

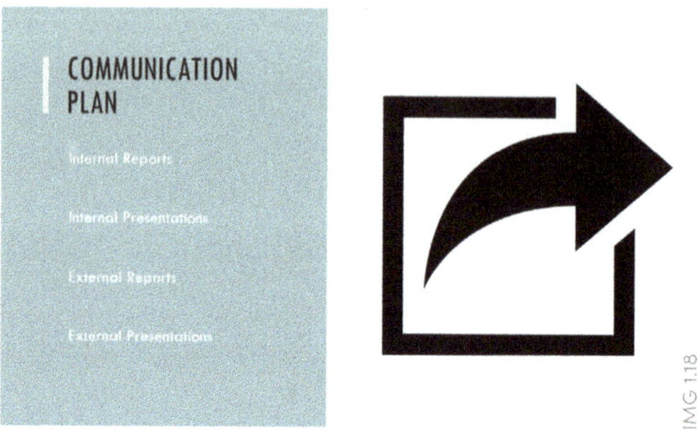

Tell stakeholders the plan to share evidence-based advice.

Slide 30: Final Slide

Evidence-based Research for Beginners– The PowerPoint Template

Presenter's name, credentials
Organization's name, location
Date of Presentation
Venue

IMG 1.19

To end the evidence story well, a final slide shows the evidence-based research title and presenter's contact information. It takes about 15 minutes to present a concise, logical evidence story.

In each remaining chapter, readers learn more details about essential skills for a basic evidence-based research project. This template is a quick tour of evidence-based research.

Reference

Aristotle. (2022). *How to Tell a Story: An Ancient Guide to Storytelling for Writers and Readers* (P. Freeman, Trans.). Princeton University Press.

Dang, D., Dearholt, S. L., Bissett, K., Ascenzi, J., Whalen, M. (2021). *Johns Hopkins Evidence-Based Practice for Nurses and Healthcare Professionals: Model and Guidelines* (4th ed.). Sigma Theta Tau International. Honor Society for Nursing.

Melnyk, B. M., Fineout-Overholt, E. (2023). *Evidence-Based Practice in Nursing and Healthcare: A Guide to Best Practice* (5th ed.). Wolters Kluwer.

Polit, D., Beck, C. T. (2017). *Nursing Research: Generating and Assessing Evidence for Nursing Practice*, (10th ed.). Wolters Kluwer.

Credits

IMG 1.1: Generated with PowerPoint. Software is Copyright © by Microsoft.

IMG 1.14a: Copyright © by Microsoft.

IMG 1.15a: Copyright © by Microsoft.

IMG 1.18a: Copyright © by Microsoft.

CHAPTER 2

Find Evidence

LEARNING GOALS

1. Differentiate between internet search engines and indexed library databases.
2. Explain the value of indexed library databases compared with internet search engines.

Smartphones have changed everything. To find a record with a smartphone, just type a word or phrase into an **internet search engine** and hit Enter. Internet search engines retrieve all related records. Four common U.S. search engines include Google, Yahoo, Edge, and Foxfire. For example, I put the phrase "diabetes mellitus" into the Google Chrome search engine. It retrieved 242,000,000 results in 0.64 seconds (see Figure 2.1).

Wow! Two hundred forty-two MILLION results! In less than one second! That was quick. But—is it efficient? Would all those records be the best evidence? Wouldn't an ethical evidence-based researcher review all 242,000,000 results to find the best evidence? In truth, quick internet searches retrieve both good and bad records. Internet search engines retrieve all. That means unfiltered, biased, even fake records mingled with actual records.

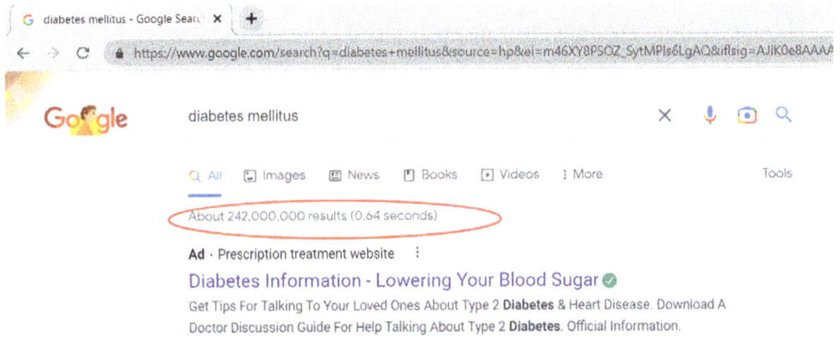

FIGURE 2.1 Screenshot of Google Chrome search for diabetes mellitus

In contrast to internet search engines, indexed library databases are choosy. Indexed databases screen journals for certain criteria before the journal is admitted to the database. When people access indexed library databases, they can retrieve scholarly, peer-reviewed articles and abstracts. As Sharma and Verma (2018) have noted, "predatory journals are not indexed in major bibliographic [library] databases, such as PubMed, Medline, Web of Sciences or Scopus" (p. 228). Predatory journals and conferences use fraud to trap naïve scholars. Predators promise quick publication of articles for a high price. The articles lack peer review. Predatory journal articles could appear on the internet. Indexed library databases guard their records from substandard, fake, or highly *biased* evidence.

Databases are either government funded, like PubMed, or privately owned, like CINAHL, ERIC, Medline, or Web of Science. Indexed databases screen journals for certain criteria before including those journals. They hold peer-reviewed articles and abstracts from scholarly journals. For example, the government-sponsored database PubMed houses about 7,000 journals with "35 million citations and abstracts of biomedical literature" (National Institutes of Health, n.d.). In contrast, CINAHL has about 1,400 journals focused on nursing and allied health (EBSCO, n.d.). The number of records retrieved from each database varies with database size.

Remember the internet search for diabetes mellitus? Hundreds of millions of records were retrieved in less than one second. Let us put "diabetes mellitus" into the U.S. government database PubMed and compare. PubMed retrieves 561,067 peer-reviewed, scholarly articles (see Figure 2.2).

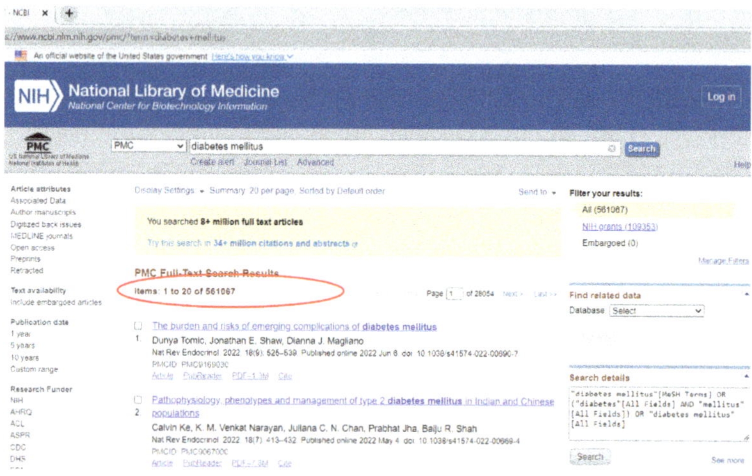

FIGURE 2.2 Screenshot of PubMed search for "diabetes mellitus"

Now search CINAHL for "diabetes mellitus." It has fewer journals than PubMed. The CINAHL search retrieves 190,774 records (see Figure 2.3).

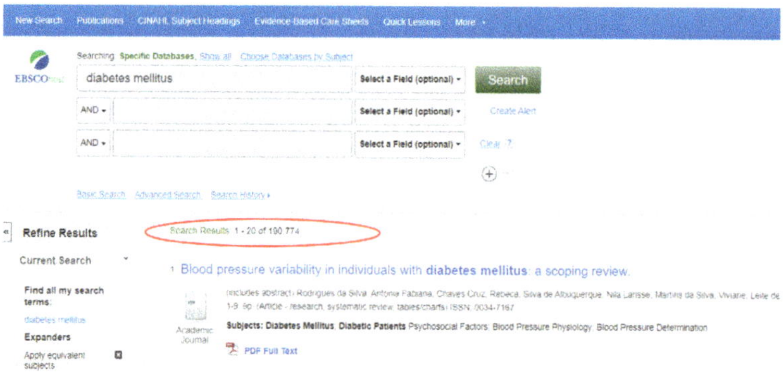

FIGURE 2.3 Screenshot of CINAHL search page for "diabetes mellitus"

To search for the best evidence means to search purposely for valid, unbiased, relevant evidence. What rises to the top of the page first in a library search is usually the most recent record. Not so for the internet. Private businesses can make deals with internet search engine companies. They can arrange for their business pages to appear first as ads with certain search terms. Look at the first entries for "diabetes mellitus" on the Google Chrome page. Do you see the ads for prescriptions? (See Figure 2.4.)

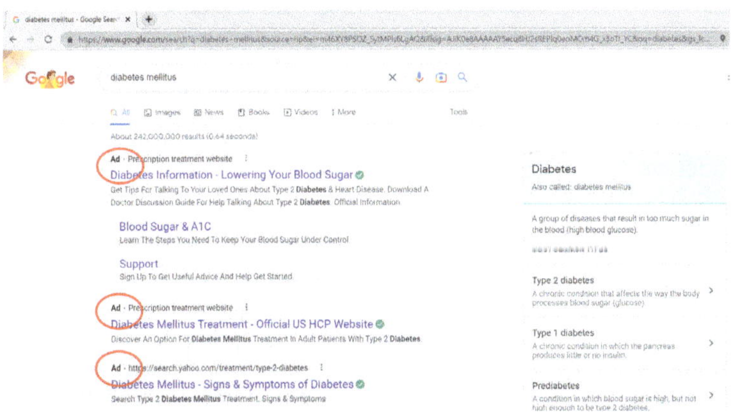

FIGURE 2.4 **Screenshot of Google Chrome search for "diabetes mellitus" with ad circled.**

Because they're so selective with the journals they index, records retrieved through library databases are more likely to be genuine. Library databases give researchers confidence that the results are valuable. In contrast, internet search engines do not assure content or quality. Records can be incorrect, misguided, fake, or purposely misleading. Anyone who uses those records can be misdirected to evidence-*biased* findings. *Biased* records defeat the purpose of evidence-based research.

What about the volume of records? Finding 500,000 records in PubMed or 170,000 records in CINAHL can overwhelm researchers. No one can read and evaluate a half million scholarly research articles in a timely manner to answer an evidence-based research question. Luckily, library databases have tools to help researchers wisely limit their results. Search tools can help researchers analyze results in an interactive way to retrieve specific records. More about the interactive analytical evidence selection process is included in Chapters 6 and 7.

Where Can Researchers Find Genuine Evidence?

Scientific research evidence appears in peer-reviewed journals as final published reports. Anyone who can read the journal can access that evidence. Quantitative research provides empirical evidence. Empirical evidence uses numerical data, observations, or facts. Qualitative researchers collect narrative data through in-depth interviews or as participant observers immersed in a culture. Research studies that use mixed methods combine quantitative and qualitative methods in a single study. That means that mixed-methods research can have numerical and narrative data.

Besides research studies, peer-reviewed journals publish a variety of **non-research evidence**, too. Experts, alone or in groups, author non-research evidence articles. When groups of experts work together, they author articles called consensus statements, white papers, or position papers. Healthcare professional experts work together to author clinical practice guidelines. For example, the American Heart Association provides clinical practice guidelines about strokes and heart attacks written collaboratively by clinical experts. To see examples of clinical practice guideline articles, go to the website of the American Heart Association. Click on "Professionals" tab. Next, under the Quality Improvement section, click on "Get With the Guidelines" link (American Heart Association, n.d.). On the next page scroll down to a variety of current clinical guidelines.

Individual experts write editorials and opinion pieces. When appraising non-research evidence based on the work of experts, researchers evaluate authors' expertise and credibility to decide if non-research evidence is worth using. Expertise might be evident from the position held by the expert. "Education" means the formal education the expert had in the field of which expertise is claimed.

One type of private non-research evidence is **internal organizational data** from **quality improvement projects**. Members of an organization might analyze internal organizational data. However, internal organizational results might remain private to the organization after the analysis.

In summary, each path to best evidence has its own unique strengths and challenges. Using internet search engines might be a way to find information in a hurry. However, that is not an evidence-based researcher's best way to find evidence. Indexed library databases offer researchers the best chance to retrieve relevant evidence.

References

American Heart Association. (n.d.) Get with the Guidelines. https://www.heart.org/en/professional/quality-improvement/get-with-the-guidelines

EBSCO. (n.d.). CINAHL Database. https://www.ebsco.com/products/research-databases/cinahl-database

National Institutes of Health. (n.d.). PubMed Overview. National Library of Medicine. https://pubmed.ncbi.nlm.nih.gov/about/

Sharma, H., Verma, S. (2018). Predatory journals: The rise of worthless biomedical science. *Journal of Postgraduate Medicine*, 64(4): 226-231.

Credits

Fig. 2.1: Copyright © by Google.

Fig. 2.2: Generated with PubMed, https://pubmed.ncbi.nlm.nih.gov/. National Library of Medicine, U.S. Department of Health and Human Services (HHS).

Fig. 2.3: Generated with CINAHL Database. Copyright © by EBSCO Information Services.

Fig. 2.4: Copyright © by Google.

CHAPTER 3

Research and Evidence-Based Research

LEARNING GOALS

1. Explain two histories of evidence-based practice.
2. Relate evidence-based research to quality improvement.
3. Grasp basic elements of the scientific research process. [AACN essential 4.1d]
4. Classify evidence as either scientific research or nonresearch scholarship.
5. Describe criteria for three categories of primary single-quantitative research studies.
6. Separate experimental, quasi-experimental, and non-experimental quantitative studies.

Two Histories of Evidence-Based Practice

One story about evidence-based practice says it began with evidence-based medicine. Archie Cochrane was a Scottish physician and statistician who studied Britain's National Health Service bills. He wanted to know which medical treatments were useful and which were not. Cochrane wanted physicians to base their advice to patients on high-quality research. He favored randomized controlled trials as the best evidence. After, Cochrane's death, his colleagues developed the Cochrane Collaboration in 1993. Under the direction of Chalmers, The Cochrane Colloboration developed criteria for systematic research reviews. They also created a way to rank levels of research evidence (Dang et. al. 2022; Greenhalgh, 2004).

Cochrane's ideas sparked Dr. David Sackett's similar efforts in Canada. Sackett defined evidence-based medicine as "the conscientious, explicit, and judicious use of current best evidence in making decisions about the care of individual patients" (Sackett, Rosenberg, Gray, Haynes, Richardson, 1996, p. 71). In 1995, Richardson and colleagues proposed the P-I-C-O question format. Between the 1970s and 2000s, physicians refined the ways to find, critically appraise, and use research to answer medical questions.

Nursing scholars adopted the P-I-C-O approach to evidence-based nursing practice in the late 1990s. Today, nursing authors Melnyk and Fineout-Overholt (2023), Dang et al. (2022), and Polit and Beck (2017) use a P-I-C-O question format. They also use a pyramid to rank levels of evidence in their EBP models. However, the levels of evidence differ from model to model. Other nursing EBP models lack PICO questions.

An Important Other History

The history of healthcare quality improvement and industrial quality research began concurrently in the early 1900s. These two movements preceded the advent of evidence-based practice by decades. Brennan and Berwick (1996) tell the history of healthcare quality improvement research and regulation in their book *New Rules: Regulation, Markets, and the Quality of American Health Care.* They explain one path to quality research called the learning tradition. In the learning tradition, people use assessment results to learn, give feedback, and change. The learning path, like total quality improvement (TQI) in business, is cyclical. Brennan and Berwick describe a second path to healthcare quality called the assessment tradition. People who use the assessment path focus on outcomes assessment to ensure compliance with standards. Both paths began at Johns Hopkins University. A third path to quality is through regulation. Regulatory laws define what is expected and permitted. Regulation protects standards. Regulation does not inspire change.

Healthcare quality research began in the United States and Europe from 1900 to 1920. In 1904, the American Medical Association created the Council for Medical Education. The council ranked medical schools by their graduates' failure to pass medical board exams. Meanwhile, the Carnegie Foundation hired Abraham Flexner to study medical education quality separately. Flexner made his report in 1910. Individual surgeons began reporting on their "end-results," or outcomes of surgeries performed, at the American College of Surgeons annual meetings (1913–1920). The intent of the reports was to inspire quality improvement in surgical techniques and to improve how surgeons taught medical students. Creation of medical education standards (1920s) led to hospital standards (1930s). Over time, standards led to regulatory efforts to uphold the standards. Today, government and private agencies conduct regulatory visits to ensure that healthcare agencies meet the regulatory standards of care.

Healthcare quality research parallels the evolution of industrial quality research. Walter Shewhart (1891–1967) and W. Edwards Deming (1900–1993) were key figures. They each examined industrial work quality. W. Edwards Deming showed that management quality affects all other aspects of work quality. Deming developed a process called Plan-Do-Check-Act. Later, Deming changed "check" to "study." Health professionals today still use Plan-Do-Study-Act theory to use evidence-based research advice.

How Evidence-Based Research Relates to Quality Improvement

The two brief histories of evidence-based practice and quality improvement above show one point. Analysis of data and evidence is key to quality improvement and evidence-based practice. The name "evidence-based practice" first occurred in the early 1990s. Nursing and medicine both credit Cochrane as the inspiration for the contemporary evidence-based practice movement . Business professionals know names like Shewhart and Deming as quality gurus. In this era of interprofessional collaborative teams, knowing how the two paths relate to each other is valuable.

Scientific Research Process—A Brief Overview

Beginners often struggle to understand scientific research. It can seem as if research is written in a private language. The truth is that experienced scientists author reports for other scientists. To be able to read and use research, beginners must learn the research language and ideas that scientists use. For example, could a novice who does not know what a variable is explain how independent variables differ from dependent variables? Or identify confounding variables? This section is about elements of scientific research language and process.

Scientific research starts with interesting, unanswered questions. Difficult issues without clear answers inspire great questions. Deeply felt gaps in knowledge that are hard to answer can inspire questions. Scientists use those ideas to write **research questions.** Concepts in research questions are often called **variables.** For **experimental** studies, quantitative researchers use **independent** and **dependent variables** to develop questions. The independent variable is the experimental intervention. The dependent variable is the expected effect or outcome of the intervention. For example, a music therapist works with post-stroke patients and wonders: "What is the effect of tailored music therapy on brain healing after stroke?" This question's intervention (the independent variable) is "tailored music therapy." The effect or outcome (the dependent variable) is "healing after stroke."

Quantitative methods use instruments to collect measurements that are statistically analyzed. Instruments can be tools such as thermometers to measure temperature, or paper and pencil instruments to measure subjective phenomena, like pain, or anxiety. Two words important to quantitative instruments are "reliability" and "validity." If a researcher measures the water temperature with an electronic thermometer, it will be important to know that the measurements are stable over time (reliable) and that the temperatures are true (valid).

In contrast, qualitative researchers collect conversational or narrative data during interviews or while being immersed in a culture. They do not use statistics to analyze narrative data. Rather, qualitative researchers examine narratives for patterns and themes. Qualitative researchers are also interested in the stability and truth of their data, so they look for characteristics such as dependability, confirmability, and trustworthiness. Even though the methods' underlying philosophy and language are different, both types of researchers are interested in the quality and interpretations of data.

Evidence-based researchers must understand that qualitative research questions use non-experimental methods to explore topics. However, even though qualitative research is non-experimental, that does not make it "nonresearch" evidence. Researchers use phenomenology to examine the essence of a phenomenon or the lived experience of a phenomenon. Grounded theory researchers study social processes. Ethnographers study cultures. A phenomenologist might ask the question: "What is the lived experience of long COVID?"

To set up primary research studies, researchers write research **purpose** statements to show the rationale and direction of the study. They write research questions in proper format. **Study aims** are specific goals researchers want to achieve with their studies. **Hypotheses** are the predicted answers to quantitative research questions. Hypotheses are only written for quantitative studies where statistical analysis can be used to accept or reject the hypothesis. Researchers combine these and other efforts to write research **proposals**.

A proposal outlines the full study, step-by-step. Research proposals must state the method and design, sampling plan, data gathering procedures, data management and analysis plans, and any other elements of that study. Researchers submit complete **research proposals** for primary studies to the institutional review board for approval. Upon approval from the institutional review board, researchers may begin their studies.

Scientific Research Categories

Scientific research includes several broad categories already mentioned, such as quantitative, qualitative, and mixed methods. Quantitative and qualitative are two categories of research with distinct philosophies and methods. The language for each category is different.

In contrast to the broad categories of quantitative and qualitative research, evidence-based research uses multiple kinds of evidence. Evidence-based researchers must learn to critically appraise different research and nonresearch evidence according to the intent, standards, and practices for each type of evidence. Three common subcategories of research evidence include the following: 1) single research studies; 2) secondary analyses of data; and 3) secondary analyses of multiple single studies. Nonresearch evidence includes scholarly articles written by experts. Chapter 8 explains these subcategories and ideas in greater detail.

Categories of Evidence

Two broad categories of evidence are 1) **scientific research evidence** and 2) **nonscientific evidence**, also called **nonresearch evidence.** Within those two broad categories, many specific types of evidence exist. Sorting the evidence correctly is important. Each type of evidence has its own criteria for critical appraisal.

Scientific Research Evidence

A common type of evidence for practice-based professions is **scientific research evidence**. Research is a systematic study that uses defined procedures to answer a question. The main goal of scientific research is to develop new knowledge. When researchers plan studies, they try to avoid bias. They conduct rigorous studies to obtain accurate, valid, reliable data. Rigorous researchers report findings with clear answers to interesting questions. In contrast, poorly conducted studies reveal signs of confusion, contradiction, or weakness. Readers must learn to assess research for rigor or weakness. Chapter 9 has more content about appraising research.

Researchers group studies by their methods. Two major categories of research methods are 1) **quantitative** and 2) **qualitative**. A third type of research, called **mixed methods**, combines quantitative and qualitative methods into a single study.

Quantitative research involves collection, analysis, and interpretation of numerical data. Single primary research studies can be either quantitative or qualitative. This beginner's guide focuses on single primary research studies to help readers learn basic ideas about research and evidence-based research skills and concepts. Books two and three present more complex content about research evidence.

Sorting research into subgroups includes primary research studies and secondary analysis studies. A **primary research** study means that researchers enroll a new sample, then collect, analyze, and interpret data. Researchers publish primary study findings in peer-reviewed articles. Usual types of primary quantitative research studies are experimental studies, quasi-experimental studies, and non-experimental studies. Common types of primary qualitative research studies are phenomenological, grounded theory, ethnographic, and historical studies.

Secondary data analysis of previously published studies has three paths. The first path is **meta-analysis**. Quantitative researchers use special statistical software to conduct a meta-analysis of previously reported research studies. Researchers compile statistics from multiple studies about one research question into a meta-analytic software program. This new study is a special statistical analysis of multiple studies. The researcher did not collect the original data and did not enroll the original samples, but used previously published statistics. Meta-analyses show the **effect size**. Researchers who want to know the strength of research about a topic want to know if the effect is strong, moderate, or weak. Meta-analysis reports are highly valued by evidence-based researchers.

The second path is **meta-synthesis**. Qualitative researchers conduct meta-syntheses of qualitative studies. They compile themes from qualitative research studies on a single topic. They analyze the themes to arrive at a broader, more encompassing theme. Two or more qualitative researchers conduct meta-synthesis together. It gives insight into the strength of qualitative evidence for that topic. Meta-synthesis reports are highly valued.

The third path is **formal systematic reviews**. Researchers conduct systematic reviews on previously published research. Systematic reviews follow strict procedures to meet the standard for systematic reviews. Researchers who are not able to perform a meta-analysis due to a lack of certain statistical data elements or who wish to combine an analysis of quantitative and qualitative studies about one research topic might engage in a formal systematic review. Unlike literature reviews, formal systematic reviews show clear search strategies with library databases. They reveal all choices to include or exclude articles. To ensure that either a meta-analysis or systematic review meets the standards, readers can use a checklist. Found on the PRISMA website (www.prisma-statement.org), the PRISMA acronym stands for Preferred Reporting Items for Systematic Reviews and Meta-Analyses. Published literature reviews are not all systematic reviews.

Finally, researchers with research doctorates use extremely large datasets, called **Big Data**, to conduct specific statistical analyses. Three examples of government Big Data sets are the U.S. national census, Medicare data, and the U.S. National Inpatient Sample.

Single Quantitative Research Studies

Single primary research studies use either **quantitative, qualitative**, or **mixed methods**. To conduct primary studies with human beings, researchers enroll a sample of volunteers, collect raw data, analyze data, and report new findings. Before seeking human volunteers for research studies, researchers must draft a full research plan called a **proposal**. The proposal goes to an **institutional review board (IRB)** for ethical review and approval. Without approval from an IRB, researchers may not conduct any study with human beings.

Quantitative Research Evidence

Single quantitative studies are well planned and controlled in advance so results will be unbiased, ethical, and relevant. The **gold standard** for single quantitative studies is **experimental research**. Another name for experimental studies is **randomized controlled trials**. Experiments or randomized controlled trials start with important unanswered questions. Experiments have three conditions: 1) an **experimental intervention**, also called a manipulation, for the experimental group; 2) a **control group** that does not receive the intervention; and 3) **random assignment** of volunteers to either the experimental or control group.

The experimental group of volunteers must be equivalent to the control group before a study begins. To be "equivalent" means that both groups should have similar numbers of volunteers with similar characteristics. For example, if the experimental group has 20 volunteers but the control group has 5 volunteers, the two groups are unequal. Unequal groups can lead to biased results. If the experimental and control groups each have 20 volunteers, but one group has children ages 3, 4, and 5 years old and the other group has children ages 10, 11, and 12 years old, the groups are not equivalent due to differences between the volunteers' characteristics. Unequal groups can lead to biased or distorted results.

Two other categories of single quantitative research studies include **quasi-experimental studies** and **non-experimental studies**. Quasi-experimental studies are not true experiments. One of three elements needed for experiments is missing. For example, random assignment of the intervention to volunteers is not possible. Instead of calling that study a randomized controlled trial, that study is either a **controlled trial** or a **controlled trial without randomization**. A more common name is **quasi-experimental study**. Ethical reasons can prevent a randomized controlled trial. When withholding an intervention from a control group is unethical, the study is quasi-experimental. When experimental and control groups are unequal, the study is called a **nonequivalent control group design**.

Researchers who conduct **non-experimental** or **descriptive** studies collect and analyze data without any intervention. Descriptive studies are exploratory. Case-control designs are retrospective. Researchers extract data from cases that have the study variable. Other non-experimental or descriptive studies collect data through surveys.

PURPOSEFUL PRACTICE EXERCISES

Go to Cognella Active Learning and use the purposeful practice exercises to check what you have learned so far.

Non-Research Evidence

Another category of evidence is **nonresearch evidence**. Nonresearch evidence can be **theoretical** or **anecdotal evidence**. Nonresearch evidence consists of experts' theories, knowledge, consensus, or experiences. Individual experts or groups of experts write nonresearch evidence articles. Nonresearch evidence is not research. In contrast, researchers collect and analyze data for non-experimental research, which lacks an experimental intervention, this is research. Non-experimental research must not be confused with nonresearch.

Individual Experts

Nonresearch evidence written by individual scholars appears in the literature as **opinion articles, op-eds, essays, letters to the editor, editorials**, or **in-depth narrative analyses of events or ideas**. Evidence-based research is based on the idea of finding a pool of unbiased, concrete research-based evidence. Individual expertise is one person's opinion in the total body of evidence.

Experts in any field can use rival theories to explain things. For example, two people can give separate expert opinions about how to motivate employees. One person might use a transformational leader theory that honors people's desires to be creative leaders. That person might urge employees to share innovative ideas. Another person might use a transactional leader style that views employees as rule followers. That person might use penalties and rewards to prompt employees to obey rules. Two experts use rival theories. Evidence-based researchers who gather evidence about how to motivate employees would include both experts' views of employee motivation. Those views are nonresearch evidence.

This example raises a question. Who is an expert? Experts must have proper credentials to confirm their expertise. Credentials can include a person's education, licensure, professional certifications, and successfully held relevant professional positions.

Non-Research Evidence Authored by Groups of Experts

The **best nonresearch evidence** is peer-reviewed reports authored by groups of experts. Examples of group-based nonresearch evidence are 1) **clinical practice guidelines**, 2) **consensus statements**, 3) **white papers** or **position papers**, and 4) **literature reviews that are not systematic research summaries**.

Experts work together to develop guidelines or statements. The authors might use research evidence, but this evidence is nonresearch. When evidence is not the report of a research study, it is nonresearch.

Organizational Contributions

Another type of nonresearch evidence is reports from **quality improvement projects**. Reporting data from quality improvement projects, either at professional conferences or in professional journals, can make it seem like quality improvement projects are the same as research evidence. The lack of institutional review board approval is a major clue that quality improvement data, even when reported in a public venue, are not research evidence but nonresearch evidence.

STUDY BOX

GET TO KNOW THE WORDS, PHRASES, AND IDEAS

Research evidence = scientific research evidence = scientific evidence

Scientific research requires care, rigor, and it can be primary or secondary.

Research evidence can be either high quality, medium quality, or low quality.

Nonresearch evidence = theoretical or anecdotal evidence = expert opinion

Nonresearch evidence is produced by individual experts or groups of experts.

Nonresearch evidence can be high quality, medium quality, or low quality.

Confidence in high-quality evidence is strong.

Confidence in medium-quality evidence is cautious.

There is no confidence in low-quality evidence, which should not be used.

Single primary quantitative research studies = controlled experiments

Randomized controlled trials = experimental research studies = quantitative

Quasi-experimental studies = controlled trials = controlled trials without randomization

Nonequivalent control group design = quantitative

Non-experimental = descriptive = quantitative or qualitative

Quantitative sampling design = large, randomized sample

PURPOSEFUL PRACTICE EXERCISES

Go to Cognella Active Learning and use the purposeful practice exercises to check what you have learned so far.

References

Brennan, T., & Berwick, D. (1996). *New rules: Regulation, markets, and the quality of American health care.* Jossey-Bass Publishers.

Dang, D., Dearholt, S. L., Bissett, K., Ascenzi, J., & Whalen, M. (2022). *Johns Hopkins evidence-based practice for nurses and healthcare professionals: Model & guidelines* (4th ed.). Sigma Theta Tau International Honor Society of Nursing.

Grant, M. J., & Booth, A. (2009). A typology of reviews: An analysis of fourteen review types and associated methodologies. *Health Information and Libraries Journal, 26,* 91–108.

Greenhalgh, T. (2004, February 4). Book Rereading of Effectiveness and Efficiency: Random Reflections on Health Services by Archie Cochrane, originally published 1978. *British Medical Journal,* 328, 529.

Melnyk, B. M., &Fineout-Overholt, E. (2023). *Evidence-based practice in nursing and healthcare: A guide to best practice* (4th ed.). Wolters Kluwer Health.

National Institutes of Health. (n.d.) Finding health statistics exercise. National Library of Medicine. https://www.nlm.nih.gov/nichsr/stats_tutorial/section4/ex7_KFF.html

Polit, D. F., & Beck, C. T. (2017). *Nursing Research: Generating and Assessing Evidence for Nursing Practice* (10th ed.). Wolters Kluwer.

Sackett, D.L., Rosenberg, W.M., Gray, J.M., Haynes, R.B., & Richardson, W.S. (1996). Evidence-based medicine: What it is and what it isn't. *British Medical Journal, 312,* 71–72.

CHAPTER 4

Research Ethics and Evidence

LEARNING GOALS

1. Explain the rationale for ethical research guidelines, including IRB guidelines (AACN 4.3a).
2. Demonstrate ethical behaviors in scholarly projects including QI and EBP initiatives (AACN 4.3b).
3. Advocate for protection of volunteers in the conduct of scholarly initiatives (AACN 4.3c).
4. Recognize the impact of equity issues in research.

Experienced scientists who conduct original research studies use the expression "the responsible conduct of research." This phrase refers to a special ethical code for researchers. The code ensures that researchers conduct studies with integrity. Researchers must respect human life and dignity for all human volunteers. The findings for ethical studies must be reported honestly and completely. The code of research ethics reflects the global scientific community's values.

People learn to conduct research from teachers, mentors, and colleagues. The elements of responsible conduct of research include data collection, management, analysis, and interpretation. It involves how volunteers are enrolled and treated. Finally, it includes research report accuracy. Yet, another side to research ethics exists—a sinister side.

Codes of research ethics aim to prevent harm to human and other living beings and to humanity and the world at large. The need for research ethics emerged during the Nuremberg Trials after World War II. The revelation of atrocities committed against human beings in the name of research shocked and outraged the global community. The Nazi program of forced inhumane treatment of human beings revealed the need to set clear limits for research. When conducted with human beings, research is a voluntary undertaking. Researchers may not force or deceive any human being to engage in any activity that leads to personal harm. Researchers must show a valid reason to conduct research. They must receive approval from an ethics committee. In the United States, the institutional review board is an ethics committee. Institutional review board members examine study proposals for research ethics concerns. Any study that is unethical is not approved. A key point in ethical research with human beings is that volunteers are enrolled after informed consent. After volunteers consent to join a research study, they may withdraw at any point and must not suffer any negative effects for withdrawing. The free will of human volunteers is upheld absolutely.

Research misconduct includes plagiarism; discovering an inadvertent or human error in one's own published research report and not reporting that error; misleading others with the report of findings; sharing or hiding research results for improper purposes, such as personal financial gain; stealing authorship from another during peer review; failing to give credit for ideas to the people who had the original ideas; hiding conflicts of interest from editors; or failing to retain research data for the standard length of time.

TABLE 4.1 Types of Scientific Research Misconduct

Data falsification
Data fabrication
Plagiarism
Finding an error in one's own published research report and not reporting that error
Manipulating research results for improper purposes, such as personal financial gain

Stealing authorship during peer review
Failing to give credit for ideas to the people who had the original ideas
Hiding conflicts of interest from editors
Failing to retain research data for the recommended length of time

Research studies published in high-quality journals undergo a rigorous peer review by colleagues. Yet, instances of journal retractions occur when questions about the studies arise. Now that research journals are online, journal editors can redact articles. They no longer exist for future readers. Before journals were in an electronic format, the only way for journal editors to reveal the discovery of misconduct was to issue a retraction statement in a later issue of the printed journal. For more in-depth information about the responsible conduct of research, readers are referred to an excellent free resource available at the National Academies Press website (www.nap.edu) called: *On Being a Scientist: A Guide to Responsible Conduct in Research.* The Committee on Science, Engineering, and Public Policy at the National Academy of Sciences, National Academy of Engineering, and Institute of Medicine of the National Academies (2009) authored this short book (Committee on Science, Engineering, and Public Policy, 2009).

Evidence-Based or Evidence-Biased?

The question "Whose evidence is this?" is not often asked when evidence-based practice research is conducted. Maybe it should be. Experienced evidence-based researchers seek the best evidence to answer their questions. How can evidence-based researchers identify research misconduct during critical appraisal to avoid adding evidence-*biased* research to their analysis?

Early in the critical appraisal of research articles, readers must check two things: 1) the journal's standing as an authentic, peer-reviewed journal and 2) the researcher's credentials. Readers are more likely to find scholarly journals within indexed library databases. Readers are at risk of finding articles from predatory journals that lack peer review if they search with internet browsers. Chapter 7 explains this issue in detail.

When screening articles to answer the PICO question, readers must check authors' credentials. Formal education and professional position must agree with the type of research report. For funded research studies, readers should check the funding agency and amount awarded. When conducting a critical appraisal of research conducted with human beings, a key piece of information is whether the study received ethical approval.

If a research report is published by someone who did not receive ethical approval or who holds an extreme or biased viewpoint, or if that report lacks a balanced consideration of all viewpoints, readers might suspect that the findings are biased. Researchers who maintain exacting standards work hard to find credible relevant evidence to show all points of view. When honest researchers refute or question a biased viewpoint, they have at least considered that the viewpoint exists. In contrast, biased researchers make little or no effort to examine all sides of a question fairly. The quality of evidence diminishes when evidence appears skewed.

Using evidence-*biased* research could harm others. *Biased* evidence usually fails to meet key criteria during critical appraisal. Since *biased* reports are not useful for evidence-based research, they are set aside as unsuitable for use.

Excellent critical appraisals, like excellent research, must be objective and careful. Novice researchers might believe all published evidence is valid and reliable. Publication is not sufficient reason to accept research reports as high quality. Critical appraisals help researchers decide whether the evidence is useful to answer the PICO question.

During critical appraisal, research misconduct might surface. While it is important to know the indicators of mistakes, negligence, and weak research, it is more important to know how to detect research misconduct attributed to devious or sly, ambitious scientists who have failed to uphold exacting standards for scientific research.

Three major categories of false or devious research reporting include 1) data fabrication, 2) data falsification, and 3) plagiarism. It is important to note that inadvertent human error is different from false or devious research misconduct. When data are reported with an inadvertent human error that might make the results seem better than they really are, someone will notice that error during peer review. Most peer reviewers kindly point out needed corrections to authors. Honest researchers value the chance to correct their reports before publication. However, if research is reported with misleading data, that misleading report can eventually create suspicion about the quality of that investigator's body of research. Once the breach of research ethics is made known to the publisher, the report will be retracted (withdrawn). Researchers can be charged with fraud.

Data fabrication is intentional. It means that researchers made up data points or results (Committee on Science, Engineering, and Public Policy, 2009). Fabricated data mislead the scientific community. Others could base their own research on dishonest reports. Once data fabrication is known, the author of fabricated research will lose his or her position, reputation, and credibility. The research study will be retracted (withdrawn) from the body of literature (Committee on Science, Engineering, and Public Policy, 2009, pp. 15–18).

The difference between data falsification and data fabrication is not easy to see immediately. Data falsification means that data were changed to give a better or more desirable outcome than the original data could provide. For example, a nutritionist recorded weekly weights for volunteers enrolled in a weight loss study. If the average weight loss in 26 weeks was four pounds but the researcher falsified the data by adding the number 2 before each person's total weight loss and made the average weight lost 24 pounds in 26 weeks, the study with nearly 1 pound per week of weight loss would look quite successful compared to the reality. In contrast, data fabrication means that a researcher who needed to enroll 350 volunteers could have enrolled 35 volunteers and then made up (fabricated) the data for the remaining 315 volunteers. No matter which part of a study is false or fabricated, the main point is that researchers who engage in misconduct engage in fraud. The example may seem extreme. It is a fake example to show how misconduct occurs.

Another example of research misconduct is falsified authorship of research articles. Authorship must be authentic. Likewise, reporting someone else's published or unpublished work as if it is one's own without citation is plagiarism. The pressure for scientists to publish frequently can entice people to engage in misconduct. That pressure is not an excuse. Misconduct is unacceptable.

Authors must include a statement about conflicts of interest. An author's conflict of interest, especially if there is a financial gain or a gain of prestige, can be another path to research misconduct. Research misconduct is not ethical. It is not acceptable. Using fake research findings can lead to irreversible harms.

In contrast to unethical researchers who engage in devious practices, ethical scientists report any limitations of their research. By the time scientists complete a research study, they are aware of their study's limitations. Sharing limitations freely is an aspect of responsible conduct of research.

Ethics, Health Equity, and Social Determinants of Health

Achieving health equity is not just a national concern in the U.S. Health equity is often tied to social determinants of health, which include factors like poverty, housing, employment, adequate food, and childhood education (National Academies of Sciences, Engineering, and Medicine, 2021). Although health equity is a long-standing international concern, the social determinants of health include social aspects beyond illnesses and health issues. The World Health Organization (WHO) was established by the United Nations in 1948 to work worldwide on global health issues (WHO, n.d.). UNESCO, the United Nations Education, Scientific, and Cultural Organization, is another division of the United Nations (UNESCO, n. d.). Its strategic objectives include addressing global social inequities by promoting development, transforming lives through education, protecting human rights, promoting inclusion and mutual understanding, protecting our global environment, and more (UNESCO, n.d.). Readers might wonder what health equity and social determinants of health have to do with evidence-based research. That question has a philosophical answer. Is the evidence for evidence-based research only the evidence that is present, or would the evidence include pieces of evidence that are missing? In the case of health and social equity, the data show that there are groups of people who lack health care, education, food, and housing. When evidence is assembled to examine any issue, whose evidence is it? Does the evidence come only from people who have health care, education, food, and housing? Or does the evidence fail to mention those aspects, also called the social determinants of health, that are the real key to improving health and social equity worldwide? In this book, collecting data to reflect the presence or absence of consideration of the social determinants of health will be addressed in Chapter 8, under the topic of developing evidence display tables.

An excellent resource to learn about social determinants of health is Chapter 2 of *The Future of Nursing 2020–2030: Charting a Path to Health Equity (National Academies of Sciences, Engineering, and Medicine, 2021)*, available to read for no cost online at the National Academies Press website (www.nap.edu). An earlier report entitled *Unequal Treatment: Confronting Racial and Ethnic Disparities in Health Care* (Smedley et al., 2003) is also available to read for no cost at the same website.

Summary

This chapter presents topics such as the responsible conduct of research, standards for research ethics, types of research misconduct, and the contrast of evidence-based research with evidence-*biased* research. This book presents a new point of view about evidence-based research. Readers see the idea that evidence is not merely what is present in each article. Evidence is also what valuable information is missing from an article. To achieve the international goal of health and social equity, truly responsible researchers today will conduct evidence-based research being informed that it is important to say which elements of data are missing from the evidence.

References

Committee on Science, Engineering, and Public Policy, at the National Academy of Sciences, National Academy of Engineering, and Institute of Medicine of the National Academies. *On being a scientist: A guide to responsible conduct in research.* National Academies Press.

National Academies of Sciences, Engineering, and Medicine. (2021). *The future of nursing 2020-2030: Charting a path to achieve health equity.* National Academies Press. https://doi.org/10.17226/25982

Smedley, B. D., Stith, A.Y., & Nelson, A. R. (Eds.). (2003). *Unequal treatment: Confronting racial and ethnic disparities in healthcare.* National Academies Press.

United Nations Education, Scientific, and Cultural Organization (UNESCO). (n.d.). https://www.unesco.org/en

World Health Organization (WHO). (n.d.). History of WHO. https://www.who.int/about/history/

PART II

Building Evidence-Based Research Skills

CHAPTER 5

Skill 1

Pose Precise PICO Questions

LEARNING GOALS

1. Grasp the basic elements of the scientific research process [AACN 4.1d].
2. Define four basic P-I-C-O question elements.
3. Explain each P-I-C-O element's sentence job (subject/noun; predicate/verb; object).
4. Explain right relationships among P-I-C-O elements.

Define Four P-I-C-O Question Elements

Evidence-based research starts with pragmatic clinical, organizational, or work-related questions about best practice. However, evidence-based researchers do not enroll human volunteers or collect new data. Evidence-based researchers seek peer-reviewed articles from indexed library databases to develop a sample of evidence. Evidence-based research questions use existing research or nonresearch evidence to answer the question. If it is available, evidence-based researchers might use internal organizational data. The P-I-C-O acronym format is used for evidence-based research questions, especially for researchers familiar with the evidence-based practice processes recommended by Melnyk and Fineout-Overholt, Dang et al., and Polit and Beck (see Chapter 3). Not all evidence-based practice researchers use P-I-C-O question formats. However, this beginner's guide uses the P-I-C-O format.

The P-I-C-O Acronym Format

The P-I-C-O acronym today is more complex than it was in 1995 when Richardson and colleagues wrote about it. Each letter in the acronym P-I-C-O can have more than one meaning. The **P** can stand for **P**atient, **P**opulation, or **P**roblem. The **I** letter can stand for **I**ntervention or **I**ssue of **I**nterest. The letter **C** usually stands for **C**omparison Intervention. It can also be a second issue of interest. The **O** letter stands for **O**utcome. To keep things simple for beginners, this book limits the meanings of the P-I-C-O elements. In this book, **P** will only mean Patient or Population, **I** will only mean Intervention, **C** will only mean Comparison Intervention, and **O** will only mean Outcome. To learn how to write a precise PICO question, it is important to be clear about each term's meaning. This structure will make it easier to learn other ideas about PICO elements.

Simple evidence-based research questions need only four PICO elements. Occasionally a fifth element is shown with the letter **T**, which stands for **T**ime Frame. The acronym format becomes PICO-T.

One key point about the value of the PICO format is that, when it is well-written, the PICO question helps evidence-based researchers focus their search strategies. When the PICO question is poorly grasped, the links between elements are misunderstood. A PICO question that lacks correct links confuses and frustrates potential evidence-based researchers.

A Concise History of How Evidence-Based Questions Got Their PICO Format

Readers might recall from Chapter 3 two pioneers of evidence-based medicine. Scottish physician and statistician Archie Cochrane (1909–1988) began writing about evidence-based practice in the early 1970s. Canadian physician David Sackett's (1934–2015) evidence-based medicine work was mainly between the 1990s and early 2000s. According to Garrett (2016), Cochrane and Sackett each posed evidence-based questions, but neither Cochrane nor Sackett posed PICO questions. Garrett states that Cochrane asked a single question: "What is the best solution to this particular health issue?" (p. 114). Twenty years later, Sackett's five-stage model of evidence-based medicine was 1) ask a question; 2) find the best evidence; 3) evaluate the evidence; 4) use evidence by applying clinical expertise and patient values; 5) evaluate. Neither pioneer used the PICO format so prevalent today.

According to Eriksen and Frandsen (2018), the PICO question format was introduced in 1995 by Richardson and colleagues to improve the quality of evidence-based medicine literature searches. Richardson et al. (1995) said that evidence-based medicine could use four basic elements: population, intervention, comparison intervention, and an outcome. This logical four-element approach to formatting evidence-based questions for physicians led to the PICO format. It was adopted by nurse scholars such as Melnyk and Fineout-Overholt, Dang and colleagues, and Polit and Beck. Although not all evidence-based researchers use it, the PICO acronym with proper links intact is valuable. P-I-C-O is now its own word—PICO.

Most people who use evidence-based research today begin by seeking research studies from library databases. This chapter unravels the first mystery of evidence-based research: how to pose precise PICO questions.

Skill 1: Pose Precise PICO Questions

The first skill for evidence-based research is to pose precise PICO questions (Stillwell et al., 2010). Well-built PICO questions are the basis for all stages of evidence-based research (Ford and Melnyk, 2019). Other skills depend on how precise and clear the PICO question is. To write strong search sentences, start with PICO words. To gather relevant evidence, use PICO words to decide on inclusion and exclusion criteria. To assemble tables that tell a direct evidence story, use PICO words to create evidence table categories.

Poorly written PICO questions strangle searches with unneeded words. That tangled path is like jogging in quicksand—people sink quickly and get nowhere fast.

Beginning evidence-based researchers might think that writing PICO questions is simple. A fill-in-the-blank template makes setting up PICO questions look easy (McClinton, 2022). If someone fills in one word for each category, what could go wrong? There is more to writing precise PICO questions than putting four words into a template. Beginners must learn how each PICO element relates to the other PICO elements. Without this understanding of "right relationship," they will pose weak PICO questions. PICO elements must be in right relationship with each other from the start for the rest of the project to flow well.

Evidence-based research models might use an algorithm to develop PICO questions. Algorithms help experienced researchers with good mentors nearby wisely refine their PICO questions. Such algorithms might be too complex for beginners to use. The algorithms' elements are not easy for people who lack research experience to use. Beginners without mentors can think they are using the algorithm correctly, even if they are not.

To become an experienced writer of precise PICO questions, it is important for beginners to start by examining how regular sentences are constructed. Once beginners understand how regular sentences are constructed, they will be able to use their sentence construction knowledge to develop strong PICO questions. So, let us start at that most basic level.

A Little Detour About Sentences (Or 15 Minutes of Fun)

Sentences are made of up words. Each word in a sentence has its own role. Each word's role forms a link with other words within each sentence. The name given to the links of words within a sentence is **syntax**. Learning about syntax for regular sentences might build basic competence about the roles and relationships that different words have. Seeing how words relate to each other in regular sentences helps evidence-based researchers write precise PICO questions. PICO elements link to each other like words in simple sentences. It takes a little time and practice to be at ease with sentence syntax. However, those efforts pay off quickly once researchers see how PICO sentence syntax is like the syntax of regular sentences.

Four types of regular sentences are declarative, interrogative, imperative, and exclamatory. Declarative sentences declare something or make a statement. They end with a period. An example of a simple declarative sentence is: "This meal is tasty."

Interrogative sentences, also called questions, seek information and end with a question mark. An example of a simple interrogative sentence, or a question: "Was that meal tasty?"

Imperative sentences give commands or orders. Imperative sentences can end quietly with a period or loudly with an exclamation point. For example, a restaurant owner can whisper a private command to the chef: "Make a tasty meal." Or a restaurant owner can loudly command the chef, "Make a tasty meal!"

Finally, exclamatory sentences usually exclaim a strongly felt emotion or idea. Exclamatory sentences always end with an exclamation point. For example, after enjoying the chef's tasty meal, a happy diner might exclaim to the waiter, "That was a tasty meal!"

Each type of sentence has its own structure and its own punctuation. Sentence structure, also called syntax, means how the words are put in order, what relationship each word has to other words in the sentence, and how word order affects the sentence's meaning.

Punctuation for regular sentences refers to symbols that tell readers to keep reading, to pause, or to stop. For example, readers stop at the full-stop points, when sentences end with a period, a question mark, or an exclamation point. Full-stop points mean that the whole idea for that sentence is complete. When an idea for the sentence is not complete, the punctuation symbol is either a comma, a colon, or a semicolon. Writers put colons into sentences when they are going to make a list of items. Listed items can be separated with commas if they are single words, or with semi-colons if the items already contain commas. When writers use commas or semicolons within a sentence, readers might pause, but they know the sentence is not complete, so they pause and keep going with the same thought. It is important to understand how punctuation works for regular sentences because evidence-based researchers write elaborate search sentences with other kinds of punctuation such as parentheses, brackets, Boolean operators and wildcards.

As noted earlier, each word has a different job to do in a sentence. The major job roles for words in sentences are 1) subjects; 2) predicates, also called verbs; and 3) objects. Subjects in simple sentences are usually the first nouns or pronouns that tell readers what the sentence is about. Nouns and pronouns are the parts of speech usually used for sentence subjects or sentence objects. Predicates in sentences are verbs or action words that tell readers what the subject is doing. Objects in sentences are the nouns or pronouns that complete the thought about what the subject is doing. If the sentence's subject produces the action (the predicate), the sentence's object receives the subject's action. This idea is key to writing clear PICO questions.

Let us examine the job roles and word parts of two simple sentences.

Birds fly. In this simple sentence, the subject is "*birds.*" The sentence is about birds. "*Fly*" is the sentence's predicate, which tells readers what action the birds are doing. Remember that the predicate is the action word. The simple declarative sentence "Birds fly" is made up of a subject and a predicate. The subject, "birds," is a noun. The predicate, "fly," is a verb, also called an action word.

The child plays. In this simple sentence, "*child*" is the subject. The sentence is about a child, and the word "*child*" is a noun. "*Plays*" is the sentence's predicate, or the action word that tells readers what the child is doing. The word "*the*" modifies "*child*." This simple declarative sentence has a subject (child), a predicate (plays), and one extra word, "the," which is called an article.

Simple sentences become more complex once an object is added. The object of a sentence is usually a noun or pronoun that completes a thought about the subject's action. Two simple sentences with objects are below.

Birds fly south. By adding the object "*south*," readers are given more information about where the birds are flying. The relationship of words in this sentence is: subject (birds), predicate (fly), object (south).

The child plays a game. By adding the object "game," readers are given more information about what the child is playing. The relationship of words in this sentence is: subject (child), predicate (plays), object (game). Two extra words, "*the*" and "a," are articles that modify the nouns that follow each article.

Sentence objects are usually the second noun or pronoun in simple declarative sentences. They complete the idea of what the subject is doing. However, objects can be made up of word phrases, such as prepositional phrases that include a noun after a preposition. Two types of sentences that people use most often in writing and speaking are declarative sentences, which make statements, and interrogative sentences, which pose questions. Each of the above examples are of simple declarative sentences. They each make a statement with a subject, predicate, and object.

Because we ask and write questions so frequently, people might think they already know how to write PICO questions. But PICO questions are not like regular questions. To build precise PICO questions word-part by word-part requires analytical skill. It is valuable to analyze regular sentences word by word first with a sentence analysis strategy called diagramming sentences. This strategy (a skill I learned as a child), will make writing precise PICO questions possible, especially when the questions are complex.

The Art of Diagramming Regular Sentences

Learning the art of diagramming regular sentences is not hard. It used to be taught to children in the fifth grade. It might now be considered old-fashioned, even obsolete (Florey, 2006). It was invented in 1877. Keep in mind that diagramming sentences is 100 years younger than ice cream (invented in 1777). If you still enjoy ice cream, maybe you will take delight in this skill.

Diagramming simple sentences can help people grasp two important types of information about words and sentences. First, as noted above, in every sentence, each word has its own job to do. The job role for a subject is different from the job role for a predicate. The job role for an object is different from the job role for an adjective or an adverb. Second, each sentence's words have a certain position in the sentence based on their job role. The sentence's subject has the vital role of telling readers what the sentence is about. The sentence's predicate has a secondary role of telling readers what the subject is doing. Finally, the object has a different role of completing the sentence's thought, since the object receives or fulfills the subject's action.

To diagram a simple declarative sentence, begin by making a horizontal line with two vertical lines. Diagram the simple declarative sentence: "The sky is blue." The subject, "sky," goes in the first box; the predicate, "is," goes in the middle box; and the object, "blue," goes in the last box. A diagram of the simple declarative sentence above looks like this:

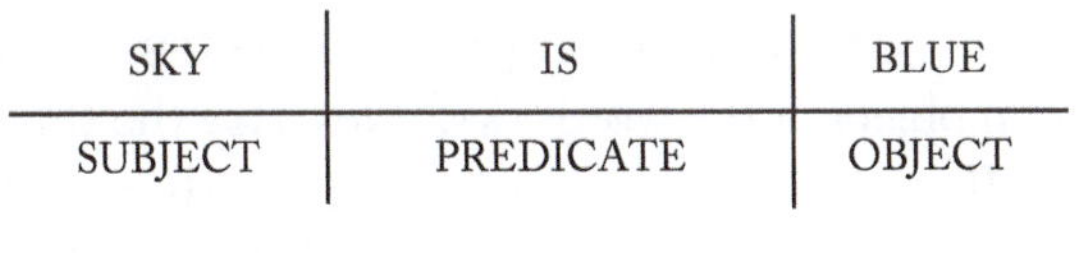

SKY	IS	BLUE
SUBJECT	PREDICATE	OBJECT

IMG 5.1

One word not written into the diagram yet is the word "*The*," which is an article that modifies the word "sky." To complete the diagram, put the word "The" underneath the word "sky" with a slanted line to show the relationship between the two words, where "The" modifies "sky."

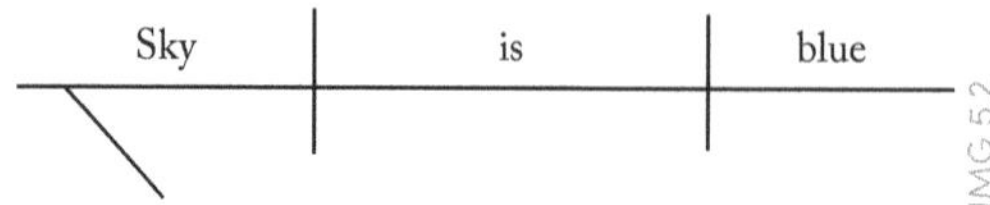

Sentence diagrams help people see how words in a sentence relate to each other. In the diagrammed sentence, the subject, predicate, and object are all clear. But what if the sentence were not so simple? What if the sentence were more complicated, with adjectives, adverbs, or other words? How would the diagram for the following sentence look?

On a mid-July morning, the sky is a soft blue color.

sky	is	blue
subject	predicate	object

IMG 5.3

To diagram this 11-word sentence, it is important to determine which word is the subject, which word is the predicate, and which word is the object. The subject of this sentence is still the word "sky." The reason I can say with confidence that the subject is "*sky*" is because the first phrase in the sentence, "On a mid-July morning," cannot stand alone and retain meaning. The sentence is about the sky, which makes "*sky*" the sentence's subject. The predicate of this sentence is still the word "is." The object of this sentence looks like it might be a word phrase: "soft blue color." However, try saying each of the three words alone after the subject and predicate. Which word fulfills the action of the subject? Let us try "sky is soft." "Soft" is not an object of the word "sky." Next, try the three words "sky is color." That phrase does not make sense either, so the word "color" is not an object. Finally, try the word "blue": "sky is blue." Yes, "blue" is the object for the subject word "sky." What are the words "soft" and "color"?

"*Soft*" is an adjective that modifies the word "blue"—"soft blue." "Soft" will go into the diagram underneath "blue" with a slanted line. Unlike the adjective "soft," "color" is not an adjective or an adverb. The word "color" is a second noun. It may go next to the word "blue" in the diagram. The first word phrase, "on a mid-July morning," is a prepositional phrase. That phrase will go into the diagram underneath the subject box. One of the most useful reasons to learn about how to diagram a sentence is that once writers can quickly see the subject-predicate-object words in a sentence, they can also see which words have more value to the sentence's meaning and which have less value. With that information, other decisions about how to write, punctuate, modify, and creatively develop a sentence are within the writer's control.

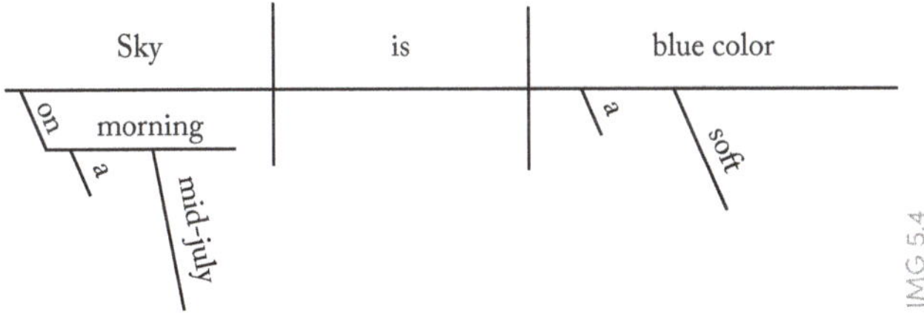

IMG 5.4

Go to Cognella Active Learning to engage in purposeful and deliberate practice exercise.

PURPOSEFUL PRACTICE

Diagram 10 simple regular sentences

DELIBERATE PRACTICE

Put together 5 PICO questions in correct format with proper word relationships based on an anecdotal problem.

PICO Syntax

To recap: In the previous section, readers saw that regular simple sentences have subjects, predicates, and objects. Subjects are usually nouns. Subjects are what sentences are about. Predicates are verbs. Predicates are the action words that show what subjects do. Objects are usually nouns that fulfill the subject's action.

Likewise, PICO questions have subjects and objects, and they have action words. In PICO language, the P word is the subject, and the O word is its object. Therefore, the P word links with the O word because the Outcome fulfills the P word's action, whether P is the Patient or the Population. That relationship between P and O parallels the link between subjects and objects in regular sentences. Subjects are linked with objects because objects fulfill subjects' actions.

PICO questions have predicates or action words. In PICO language, the I word is an action word linked with the C word, another action word. Together the I and C terms form the PICO's action. That relationship is like the predicate in a regular sentence. The predicate is the subject's action.

The value of learning how to diagram regular sentences is in knowing how that knowledge relates to PICO questions. These few rules about PICO relationships are firm. One rule is that P must link with O, because the outcome will fulfill the subject's action. Another rule is that the I word links with C, because together the Intervention and the Comparison Intervention are the action words, or the predicate, of the PICO question. Violating either of these two relationship rules will not only ruin the PICO question, it will derail the search for evidence that depends on a precise PICO question.

In the first paragraph of this chapter, PICO was defined according to the acronym's meanings. Of course, it is important to know that P can equal Problem or Population or Patient. It helps to know that the I stands for Intervention or Issue of Interest, and that C equals Comparison intervention. It is also important to know that O equals the Outcome. However, a crucial point about PICO elements is which elements are subjects, which are predicates, and which are objects when PICO questions are developed. This is the first place in the evidence-based research process where people can get confused.

Remember from Chapter 2 that the original PICO question format came from physicians who wanted to develop an efficient way to conduct literature searches for evidence-based medicine.

When Richardson and colleagues, who were all physicians, proposed the first PICO format, they designated P to stand for Patient. Since 1995, evidence-based research has moved beyond the field of medicine into other clinical and nonclinical disciplines. Others who want to engage in evidence-based research might not have "patients." So, P as it is now construed can be about patients or a population or a problem. Whatever has been the P element of PICO questions in the past could have been thought of as the subject. If physicians practiced medicine as a patient-centered profession, then P as Patients would always be the subject, or the command center, of the PICO question. Since the Intervention and Comparison Intervention are actions, the link of I with C provides a predicate for each PICO question. Finally, the O term, which means Outcome, is the object of the PICO question, which fulfills the subject's action. Therefore, P must always link with O.

To summarize, PICO questions have syntax just like regular sentences do. Having a good grasp of PICO syntax is valuable for creating precise PICO questions. The next chapter shows how to use words from precise PICO questions to build strong search sentences. Now that you've taken this detour, I hope the next time you enjoy ice cream, you will think fondly of the day you learned about sentence diagramming. 😊

References

Eriksen, M. B., & Frandsen T. F. (2018). The impact of Patient, Intervention, Comparison, Outcome (PICO) as a search strategy tool on literature search quality: A systematic review. *Journal of the Medical Library Association, 106*(4), 420–431.

Florey, K. B. (2006). *Sister Bernadette's barking dog: The quirky history and lost art of diagramming sentences.* Melville House Publishing.

Ford, L. G., & Melnyk, B. M. (2019). The underappreciated and misunderstood PICOT question: A critical step in the EBP process. *Worldviews of Evidence-based Nursing, 16*(6), 422–423.

Garrett, B. (2016). Nonresearch evidence: What we overlook but shouldn't. In M. Lipscomb, *Evidence-based practice: Debates and challenges* (pp. 113–131). Routledge.

McClinton, T. D. (2022) A guided search: Formulating a PICOT from assigned areas of inquiry. *Worldviews on Evidence-Based Nursing, 19*(5), 426–427. https://doi.org/10.1111/wvn.12598

Richardson, W. S., Wilson, M. C., Nishikawa, J., & Hayward, R. S. (1995). The well-built clinical question: A key to evidence-based decisions. *ACP Journal Club, 123*(3), A12–3.

Stillwell, S. B., Fineout-Overholt, E., Melnyk, B. A., & Williamson, K. M. (2010). Evidence-based practice step-by-step: Asking the clinical question: A key step in evidenced-based practice. *American Journal of Nursing, 110*(3), 58–61.

Credits

CHAPTER 6

Skill 2

Build Search Strategies

LEARNING GOALS

1. Translate P-I-C-O elements into "close cousin" search terms, avoiding synonyms.
2. Demonstrate "right relationship" among P-I-C-O words.
3. Use an interactive analytical approach to search databases with proper commands.
4. Analyze subject major headings to find close cousin search terms.
5. Use analysis of subject major headings to refine inclusion and exclusion criteria.
6. Screen articles to establish the final set of evidence

Translate P-I-C-O Elements into Close Cousin Words (Avoid Synonyms)

The skill of building effective search strategies starts with precise PICO questions. Each P-I-C-O word informs separate layers of the search strategy. The idea that P-I-C-O words must be in "right" relationship continues in this chapter. The right relationship of P terms with O terms is vital to the P and O search layers. This search layer unites the subject with the object. Likewise, the right relationship of I terms with C terms is key to building the search strategy layer for actions: the interventions. For evidence searches to be effective, each multilayered search needs more than one search word for each P-I-C-O word. Wise researchers pair each P-I-C-O term with close cousin words.

The phrase "close cousin words" means practical alternative research words. Close cousin words are different from synonyms. The idea of seeking synonyms can mislead beginners about how to find the right extra words for an effective search. Yet, evidence-based practice textbooks often call alternative search words "synonyms." By definition, a synonym is any word with a similar meaning to another word. In everyday language, people often use synonyms to express ideas. It is easy to find synonyms in a thesaurus. However, easy access to alternative words does not make those words effective search terms. Researchers do not use *all* words to describe their findings. They choose specific, accurate, neutral words. Those choices restrict the number and the nature of alternative words that can be close cousin words.

To select useful close cousin words, researchers must ask two questions. First, how do close cousin words relate to the original PICO words? Second, how likely is it that other researchers who did not use the exact PICO words would use those close cousin words in research articles? The goal is to find close cousin words that other researchers would use in place of the exact P-I-C-O words.

For example, consider a researcher with the P (population) word "neonates." The definition of the word "neonate" is an infant in the first four weeks of life. A close cousin term for neonates might be "infants." Although the word "children" is a synonym, that word is not specific to the first four weeks of life. Children are usually older than four weeks. The search word "children" is too broad. "Children," as a synonym, does not accurately match the P word "neonates." To find close cousin terms, think the way a researcher who studies that topic might think. Try to use words that other researchers use (see Figures 6.1 and 6.2 below).

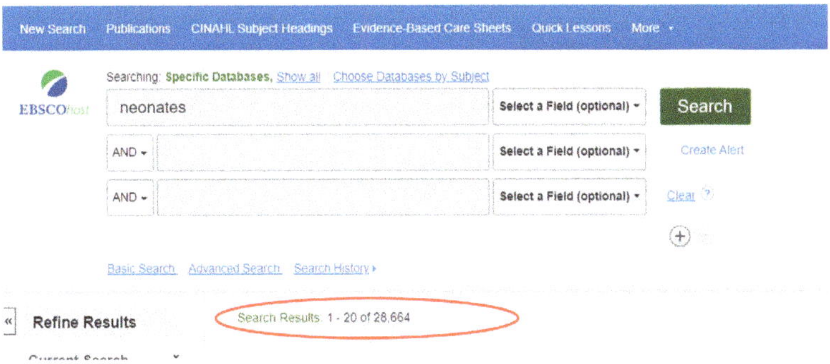

FIGURE 6.1 Results for the search term "neonates" yield 28,664 records in CINAHL.

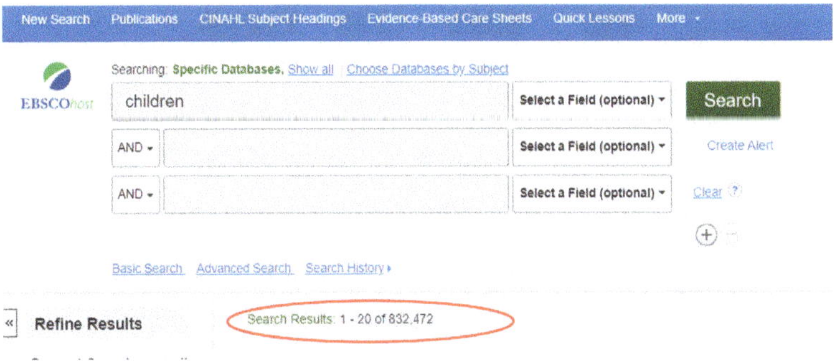

FIGURE 6.2 Results for the search term "children" yield 832,472 records in CINAHL.

Compare the two search results above. The search results for the P term "neonates" yield nearly 30,000 records. The search results for the synonym "children" yield nearly 1,000,000 records. Researchers who use a thesaurus to find close cousin words must be choosy (see Figure 6.3).

The list of synonyms below shows that most synonyms are not suitable to report on research with neonates. Words like "babe," "bambino," "dumpling," "kid," "nipper," "suckling," "tad," and "tot" are not words that scholars use to describe research results. The few synonyms that relate to neonates might be words like "baby" and "newborn." More than half the synonyms in that *Thesaurus.com*

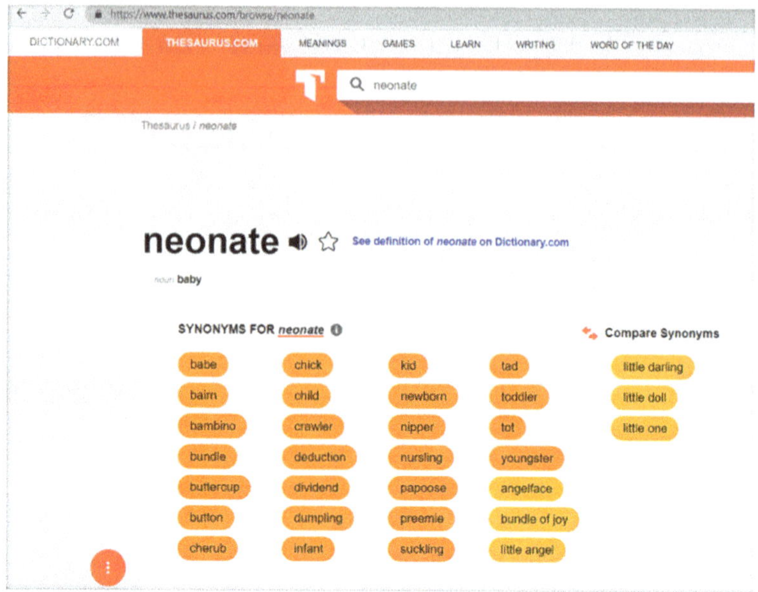

FIGURE 6.3 Screenshot of synonyms for "neonate" from *Thesaurus.com*

list are slang terms. Scholars do not use slang in research reports. Researchers would not use the word "preemie" to describe findings about neonates. Yet, the synonym "preemie" might prompt a researcher to use the word "premature" in a search.

This is where the struggle to construct an effective search strategy can increase. Search strategies start with precise PICO words. Next, P-I-C-O words prompt searches for close cousin words that other researchers might use instead of the exact PICO words. Close cousin words join the PICO words in search phrases. Sometimes, researchers build a single search sentence and use the exact sentence to search each library database. This book does not use that strategy. Instead, this book shows an interactive analytical search strategy. With an interactive analytical approach, researchers use a variety of efforts to construct the search for evidence.

An Interactive Analytical Approach to Evidence Searches

Once researchers have clear ideas for their P-I-C-O and close cousin words, they are ready to search in library databases. To give commands to a database is a complex process. Researchers need an in-depth grasp of each library database's commands and rules. The content about database rules appears in Chapter 7. This chapter explains the theory and shows the process of an interactive analytical approach.

Researchers start by putting search words into the database search screen.

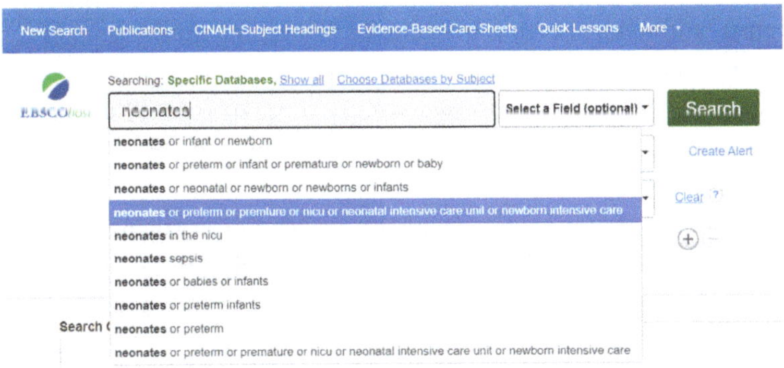

FIGURE 6.4

The figure above shows the CINAHL search screen. After typing the first P word, "neonates," into the search screen, a pull-down menu appeared. Selecting the blue highlighted choice returned 85,362 results, as shown in Figure 6.5 in the red circle.

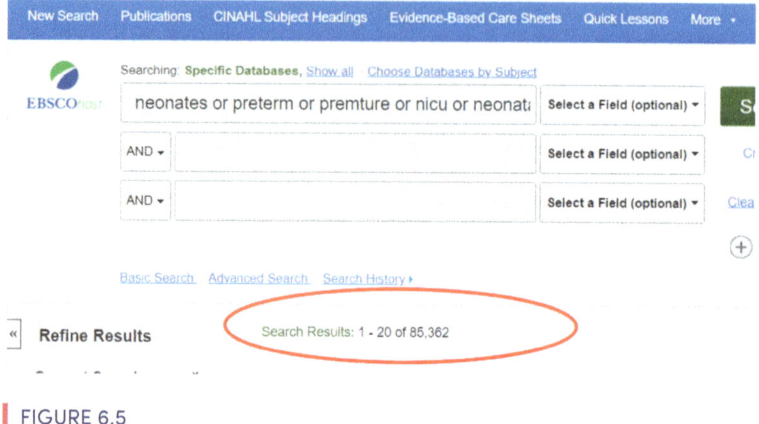

FIGURE 6.5

During the search, researchers use filters, limits, Boolean operators, and wildcards to find evidence. Searching for evidence is not a single effort. While the search is underway, researchers record all their search efforts and decisions. Keep notes in a chart like the one on the next page (Table 6.1). When presenting the final findings, researchers report the path they took to find evidence.

Table 6.1 contains data from search decisions shown in images below. A record of the decision making used with an interactive analytical approach is in each column. Comments for each decision are in the last column.

The first decision according to Table 6.1 above was to add the filter for English language. After adding that filter, CINAHL shows 83,169 results. The next choice is to filter all records for peer-reviewed scholarly journals only. The results of this choice are 76,228 articles.

TABLE 6.1 Table Used to Record Searches, Search Decisions, and Results

DATABASE: CINAHL	Date/Time June 2023		# Hits	Time Span of Publications	Decision
Key words	Close cousin words	Boolean Operators			
Neonates	Preterm Premature NICU Neonatal intensive care unit Newborn intensive care	None	85,362	1937–2023	Add filter: English language only
Neonates	Preterm Premature NICU Neonatal intensive care unit Newborn intensive care	None	83,169	1937–2023	Add limit: scholarly, peer-reviewed journals
Neonates	Preterm Premature NICU Neonatal intensive care unit Newborn intensive care	None	76,228	1937–2023	Examine Subject Major Headings Select "mothers" and "parents" from the Subject Major Headings dialog box
Neonates **+ Mothers** **+ Parents**	Preterm Premature NICU Neonatal intensive care unit Newborn intensive care	None	2,567	1947–2023	Add: AND Discharge Teaching
Neonates **+ Mothers** **+ Parents**	Preterm Premature NICU Neonatal intensive care unit Newborn intensive care	AND Discharge teaching	655	1977–2023	Re-select English to adjust the new set of articles

In the figure below (Figure 6.6), it is possible to see the number of results, the filters, and the range of publication dates.

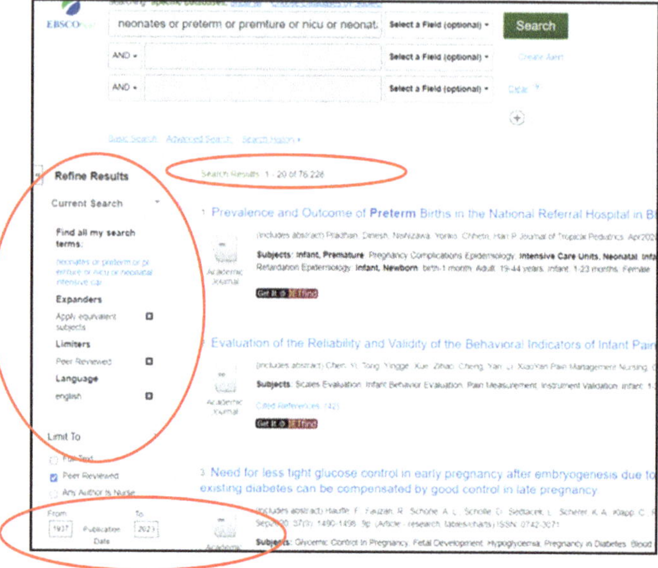

FIGURE 6.6

The results range from 1937 to 2023. Note the filters and the date range are located on the left side of the CINAHL screen. Why is it important to see the range of publication dates in this first analysis? Why not just lop off all the journal articles that were published more than 5 years ago, since evidence-based research uses only recent evidence? Experienced people with a different philosophy might trim their literature results from the start by searching only for the last 5 years of articles. That strategy is not compatible with the interactive analytical approach used in this book. This approach uses each element of information for analysis. Look at Figure 6.6. People were writing about neonates as far back as 1937. Since 1937, this result shows that there have been 76,228 peer-reviewed scholarly articles written in English. The limits are listed on the left side of the image: Limiters: Peer Reviewed; Language: English.

Now it is time to examine subtopics within these 76,228 articles. The next decision recorded in Table 6.1 is "Examine subject major headings." To examine subject major headings, go to the left side of the CINAHL page and scroll to the "show more" blue words in the Subject Major Headings filter. A gray dialog box appears, as shown below (Figure 6.7). This process will be shown again in detail in the next chapter. For now, relax and learn about the steps in the process, not the exact clicks to make.

Subject: Major Heading

Name	Hit Count
infant, premature	11,722
childbirth, premature	6,533
intensive care units, neonatal	5,313
pregnancy outcomes	3,645
intensive care, neonatal	2,611
infant, premature, diseases	2,444
pregnancy complications	2,181
infant, very low birth weight	1,985
labor, premature	1,785

Update Cancel

FIGURE 6.7

From this dialog box, it is possible to scroll down to see the major subjects for the 76,228 articles and to select segments of articles from this group of results. The researcher wants to find evidence about teen parents of premature babies. The researcher is interested in knowing if premature babies discharged to teen parents are rehospitalized within 30 days of discharge. Once the subtopics of "mothers" and "parents" are selected, that choice reduces 76,228 results to 2,567 results. An interesting thing occurred with the new group of results. The years of publication changed from 1937–2023 to 1947–2023. This means that the first article written about mothers or parents of neonates was in 1947. Ten years of articles were excluded with that search choice. Researchers know that the body of evidence is closer to answering the full PICO question. The next decision in Table 6.1 is to add a second search term about discharge education. This term goes into the second search line with the Boolean operator AND. (Chapter 7 covers Boolean operators in detail.) This new choice brings the results to 655. It also reduces the date range for publications to 1977–2023. See Figure 6.8 below.

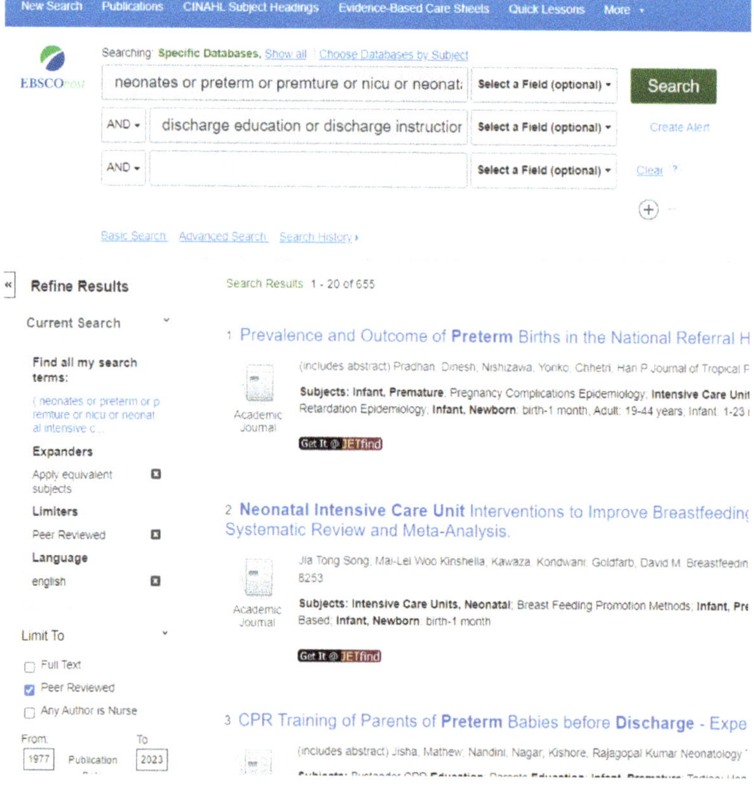

FIGURE 6.8

With this result, 30 years of articles fall away. Again, researchers who use this interactive analytical approach are confident that the evidence they need about neonates, parents, and discharge teaching did not exist earlier than 1977. These are key pieces of information to know about the data.

What Weakens Searches?

It is important for evidence-based researchers to know which choices weaken search strategies. Poorly selected major terms can make a search more difficult than it should be. For example, if a researcher who wants to study neonates uses an inaccurate word, such as "pediatrics," as a major search term. The word "pediatrics" is too broad. "Pediatrics" usually refers to patients from neonates to age 18 years. In CINAHL, the single word "pediatrics" brought up more than 220,000 results. It would be time-consuming to scan 220,000 article titles to find all relevant articles about neonates. Broad, all-inclusive terms do not help an evidence-based search. They should not be used.

Another choice that weakens search sentences is when acronyms are used instead of words. For example, a researcher wants to study Native Americans and uses the acronym AI, which can stand for American Indians. The researcher uses the following search structure: (Native Americans or American Indians or AI). What a surprise to see that a good portion of AI articles are about artificial intelligence and artificial insemination! Search engines use the exact commands that researchers give to search the entire database. If the AI acronym is used, the database might return articles about Native Americans, artificial intelligence, and artificial insemination, since it will obey the commands exactly.

Another thing that can weaken a search for evidence is when researchers place unwise or mistimed database limits on their search. Limits that are placed too early in the search process or that are too severe can reduce search effectiveness. Chapter 7 covers how to use database limits.

Finally, databases might offer a filter to retrieve FULL-TEXT articles only. This filter is a true *no-no!* for evidence-based researchers. When the search engine filters the database with FULL-TEXT, it will only provide titles and abstracts for articles that are FULL-TEXT articles. The filter could cause search engines to bypass excellent articles that do not have full-text permission but that can be retrieved another way. The goal of evidence-based research is to obtain a complete set of relevant evidence, to review the evidence, and to develop advice based on that evidence. It is crucial for researchers to know of all relevant articles.

Screening Evidence

The first search leads researchers to screen article titles, abstracts, and author credentials, to decide which articles must be retrieved. Once the most relevant articles are identified during the screening process, investigators can focus on article retrieval. Full-text articles are not used for initial screening procedures. However, if an article is deemed worthy of full critical appraisal based on its title and abstract and it is not immediately available in full-text format, investigators must retrieve the article another way. Most libraries offer an interlibrary loan service. After screening and retrieving relevant articles, the next step is to critically appraise each retained article.

An Iterative Search Process Using a Sample PICO Question

The search process itself can be used in a back-and-forth (iterative) way. This **iterative** process helps refine the final search. Researchers have a variety of ideas about which filters and limits to place during the search process. My favorite approach is to take time to develop the best grasp of the available literature before cutting any literature away. Being aware of the body of literature helps investigators make wise decisions about how to adjust the search. For example, by setting a time limit last, not first, results remain intact with each step of the search. That means that as researchers narrow the search using their exact search terms, they would see the range of publication years change. When arriving at the final set of search terms, with all other filters and limits placed, it might not be necessary to put a 5-year limit. However, as articles are trimmed away with different search terms, researchers will know where in time literature for a topic was widely or sparsely produced. Let us examine a PICO question as noted below.

In neonates born to teenage parents, how does patient discharge planning with community support compared with standard patient discharge planning affect readmissions within 30 days after discharge?

In this question, the following major search terms are P = neonates born to teen mothers; I = discharge planning with community support; C= standard discharge planning; O = readmissions; T = within 30 days after discharge.

The best way to set up this search sentence for CINAHL is:

(Neonate* or infant* or newborn*) AND (teen or teenage* or adolescent or emancipated minor) AND (parent* or mother* or mom* or dad* or father*) AND (discharge instruction* or discharge education or discharge teaching) AND (community support or ambulatory or home health) AND (readmi* or recidivism)

Note that the asterisk is used to permit CINAHL to search for singular and plural terms, for example: neonate or neonates. Note that the word "readmi*" was truncated to permit CINAHL to search for "readmission," "readmitted," and "readmit." Using the first search terms on the first three search lines, there were 2,920 articles from 1963 through 2023 (searched on March 13, 2023). Adding a fourth search line for "readmi*" brought the search results down to three articles and reduced the chronology of publications to 1990–2010. Since the search was conducted in March 2023, that chronology shows that there have been no relevant articles in the last 13 years. One question: Is this no longer a problem? Let us look at the three results.

Result 1

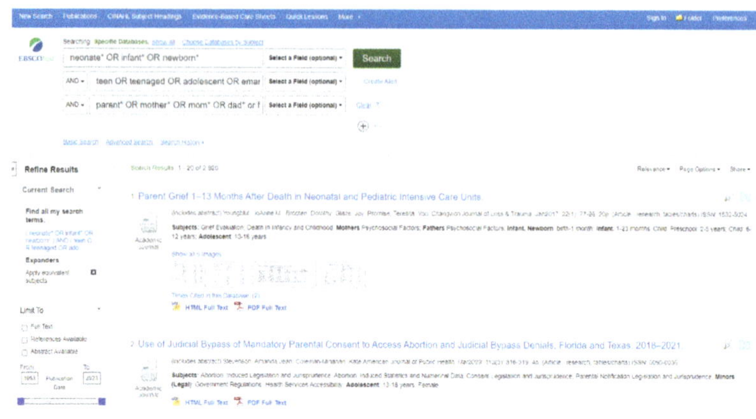

FIGURE 6.9

Result 2

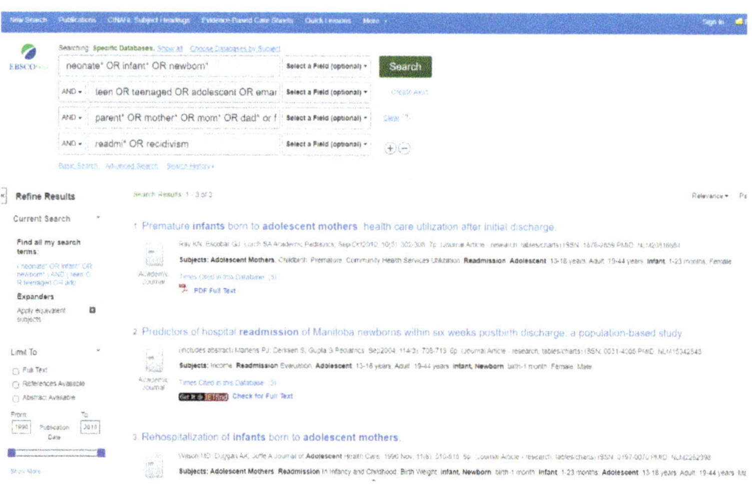

FIGURE 6.10

To make a careful study of all articles that were reduced from 2,920 to three, it is important to eliminate the last search line [readmi* OR recidivism] and examine the 2,920 articles through the filters. The first limits to be placed are "scholarly journals" and "English language." These two limits reduce the number of results to 2,538.

Result 3

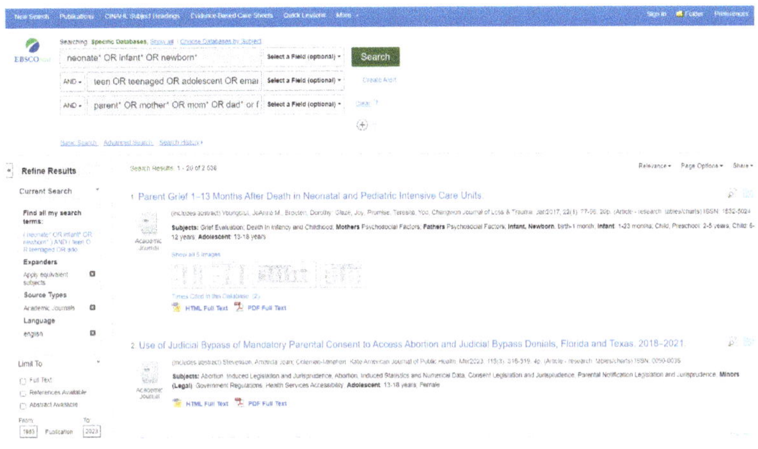

FIGURE 6.11

Next, use the subject major headings to examine what subtopics there are within those 2,538 articles. The selected subheadings were "child abuse," "premature infant," "infant care," "risk assessment," "child welfare," and "health services accessibility." Although these filters reduced the full set to 234 results, they are not helpful or relevant to the PICO question. It is time to revise the search strategy. To obtain truly relevant evidence, this search might need to be simplified.

After simplifying the search terms, CINAHL returned six results from 1990 to 2015. A quick examination of abstracts for these six articles shows that they each contain useful information to answer the PICO question. These six articles are relevant for this evidence-based research.

Result 4

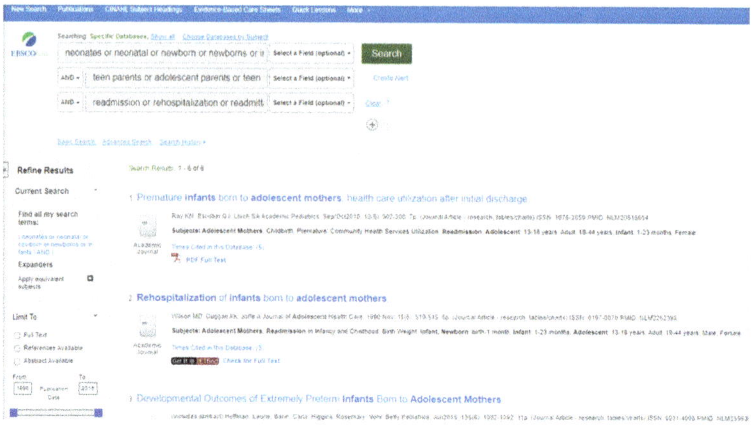

FIGURE 6.12

Of the six articles, four are from the United States (Los Angeles [2000], Philadelphia [2010], Rhode Island/North Carolina [2015], and unknown location in USA [1990]), one is from Canada (2004), and one is from Helsinki (2008). This first glance gives a brief overview of when and where the research was conducted. This list and the article publication dates prompt a question: Is it true that no one has studied readmissions of neonates born to teen mothers in the past 8 years? If so, this topic has little recent evidence. The topic might need more research.

Given that there are only six articles to critically appraise to answer this question, the next step would be to obtain each of the articles. Critical appraisal is discussed in detail in Chapter 8.

Conclusion

When building strong search strategies, it is important to start with precise P-I-C-O words. Extra search terms to find evidence must be well-chosen close cousin words, not just any synonyms. The best words are put into database search screens with correct

Boolean operators, punctuation, limits, and filters. It is wise to leave the results intact as long as possible before removing articles from before the last 5 years. The "publication year" filter helps researchers analyze that information during an iterative search process. This layered search strategy helps evidence-based researchers examine the literature carefully. If researchers continually analyze the results, they will learn to make informed choices to reduce the body of evidence to the most relevant evidence.

Credits

Fig. 6.1–6.2, 6.4–6.12: Generated with CINAHL Database. Copyright © by EBSCO Information Services.

Fig. 6.3: Generated with Thesaurus.com. Copyright © by Dictionary.com, LLC.

CHAPTER 7

Skill 3

Select Evidence

LEARNING GOALS

1. Demonstrate how to search for evidence with library databases.
2. Separate search terms from stop words to improve search results.
3. Use search filters and limits properly to exclude irrelevant articles.
4. Use Boolean operators properly.
5. Analyze subject major headings and MeSH headings to titrate the best close cousin terms.
6. Write strong search sentences with proper format.
7. Keep a record of all search strategies used for the final report.

Building a strong search for evidence requires two things: 1) knowing which search words to use and 2) knowing how each database works. Chapter 6 showed readers an interactive analytical approach to finding close cousin words and search terms. This chapter informs readers about the practical aspects of using library databases.

Search for Evidence with Library Databases

Most library databases operate in similar ways. Yet, each database has its own content focus and unique search rules. Three aspects to know about library databases are 1) the number of journals each database has, 2) how often each database is updated, and 3) which rules to use when searching for articles.

It is vital to know that individual library databases sit on large research platforms. In the United States, three major research platforms are OVID, EBSCOhost, and ProQuest. Platforms host multiple databases. When libraries purchase research platform packages, the packages include a variety of individual databases grouped together to meet each library's unique needs. Let us explore the three research platforms noted above.

Wolters Kluwer publishing offers OVID as a research database platform. OVID databases focus on medical and healthcare research. Two key journals found in OVID include the digital versions of *New England Journal of Medicine*, and *American Journal of Nursing*. OVID also offers the Joanna Briggs Institute, an Australian nursing evidence-based practice database. OVID's database collections focus on behavioral health, diversity/equity/inclusion, evidence-based health, and public health. OVID's individual databases focus on specific disciplines such as physician assistants, medical and allied health, medicine, anesthesia, pharmacy, nursing, dentistry, food science and nutrition, veterinary and animal science, and more. (WoltersKluwer, n. d.)

EBSCOhost, like OVID, has multiple individual databases dedicated to healthcare. However, EBSCOhost has a variety of individual databases that address disciplines such as art and architecture, education, business/economics/finance, communication/speech disorders, earth/environment, general news, history/political science, literature/modern languages, math and computer science, physical education, psychology/sociology/anthropology, and social work/gerontology. (EBSCOhost, n. d.)

Like EBSCOhost, ProQuest has a variety of individual databases. However, ProQuest might be the largest of the three research database platforms. According to its webpage, ProQuest has more than 450,000 e-books and streaming videos. ProQuest "encompasses 90,000 authoritative sources, 6 billion digital pages and spans six centuries" (ProQuest, n.d.). Each of the three database platforms provide individual database packages for libraries to purchase. Ask librarians which database platforms and individual databases are available at a specific library.

When people first learn to search library databases, they might be taught to search multiple individual databases at the same time by using a search screen for the entire database platform. Readers who learned that method must now transcend that search habit. Retrieving countless articles by searching multiple databases together weakens evidence-based research. When telling the evidence story, researchers must show their detailed search strategy and results for each database. That is why researchers search one database at a time. The best way to select a database is to choose one with content that matches the PICO question.

A Quick Look at CINAHL

An EBSCOhost database to examine is CINAHL, the **C**umulative **I**ndex to **N**ursing & **A**llied **H**ealth **L**iterature. This database began in print format in the 1960s. It was moved to an electronic format in 1984. Currently, CINAHL holds about 4,000,000 records from 1,400 journals. CINAHL indexes nursing and allied health journals such as nutrition, physical therapy, speech therapy, and respiratory therapy. CINAHL includes a few physician's journals. A companion EBSCOhost database called Medline indexes medical journals. Of note, CINAHL is available in 20 separate versions. It is priced accordingly. Nurses who belong to Sigma Theta Tau International Nursing Honor Society may purchase an individual monthly subscription to CINAHL. Certain versions of CINAHL offer PDF, full-text, and electronic links to journal articles. The scope of what each version of CINAHL offers differs from library to library. It depends on the package each library has purchased.

Tips for Using CINAHL

Once a single search term is entered or even partially entered, CINAHL's database might suggest more search terms in automatic drop-down menus. Researchers can examine and select these close cousin terms. This CINAHL feature makes good searches easier. However, beware of any words in the suggested terms that do not match the main PICO ideas. Prune irrelevant words to avoid retrieving unneeded information.

Another feature of CINAHL and other databases is that researchers can truncate search terms with an asterisk. For example, if a researcher wants articles about nurses, the search term "nurses" could be truncated to its core element with an asterisk, such as "nurs*" (see Figure 7.1 below). This partial word with an asterisk leads to a drop-down menu with word suggestions. Depending on the full PICO question, the researcher might select from that drop-down menu to increase the scope of the initial search.

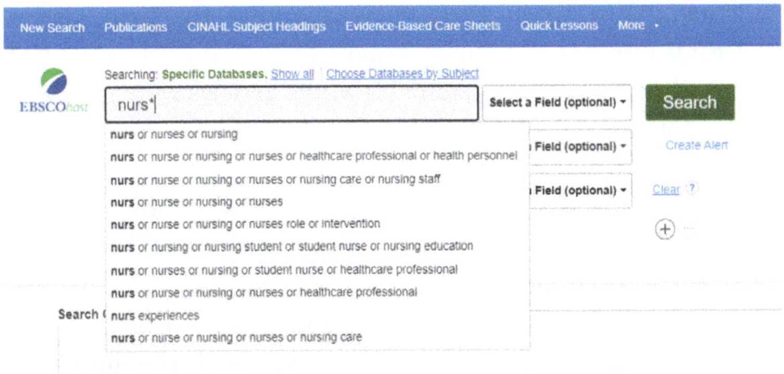

FIGURE 7.1 CINAHL recommends possible like search terms in a drop-down menu.

Isolate Search Words from Stop Words to Improve Searches

CINAHL's database has a feature called "stop words," which are articles, pronouns, and prepositions. When stop words and search terms are put into the search screen together, the database will be "stopped." The database will not be able to retrieve any research articles. Examples of words called articles are "the," and "a." Examples of words called pronouns are "she," "he," and "they." Examples of words called prepositions are "about," "above," "before," "for," and "of." A large variety of preposition words exist to set off prepositional phrases in sentences. If any stop words are used to search, CINAHL will not return any results until stop words are removed.

Use Search Filters and Limits Properly

When CINAHL returns search results, it shows the time range for years of publication on the left side of the page. Beneath that time range are two sets of filters. The first filters are **source type**, such as academic journals, dissertations, continuing education units, and magazines. Beneath that is a second set of filters: geography, age, subject major headings, gender, publications, publisher, and language. Each filter can be opened to show specific data. When researchers open each filter, they will see how the total number of articles breaks down into subcategories. Researchers can see the countries where articles were published (geography) or which age categories are contained in the set of articles. They will know the full scope of time when all articles for that topic were published. The gender filter at present breaks articles into male and female. The "publication filter" can be used to examine the exact journals where publications are located and the number of results each journal contributes. The "publisher filter" lists the publishers of the journals, with the number of results from each publisher listed. The publication and publisher filters are discussed in books two and three with the topics of systematic review and meta-analysis. Two other filters are for language, and subject major headings.

The language filter can be one of the earliest filters used during a search, especially if researchers are only able to search in a single language. In this book, English language will be set as an early filter in any searches. However, if any evidence-based research team members speak other languages, such as Spanish or Portuguese, the team member who speaks that other language might want to conduct a separate search to find articles with only that other language. When the language filter is used properly, the database reduces the results, which will include only the selected language.

One important filter in CINAHL is the subject major heading filter. It is valuable because it doubles as an analytical tool. In CINAHL, subject major headings are the database's controlled vocabulary. Keywords that authors select for their articles become subject major headings. If inexperienced authors put in weak keywords for their articles, researchers cannot find those articles easily. The database uses the terms placed into search screens to find a match in its metadata. This means that databases search for words within article titles, abstracts, listed keywords, or text.

What is interesting about the filter called "subject major headings" is that researchers can examine the list of all subtopics listed for that subject major heading. After opening the subject major headings filter, researchers can scroll down and click on the blue words "show more." This click brings up a dialog box. CINAHL's dialog box shows each major subtopic for all the results in that search. Each subtopic has the number of articles on the right side and a tick box on the left side. The next two images show results from a CINAHL search for the phrase "moral distress." That search returned 1,886 articles with a publication time span of 1987– 2023. The next image is of the dialog box for the subject major heading filter.

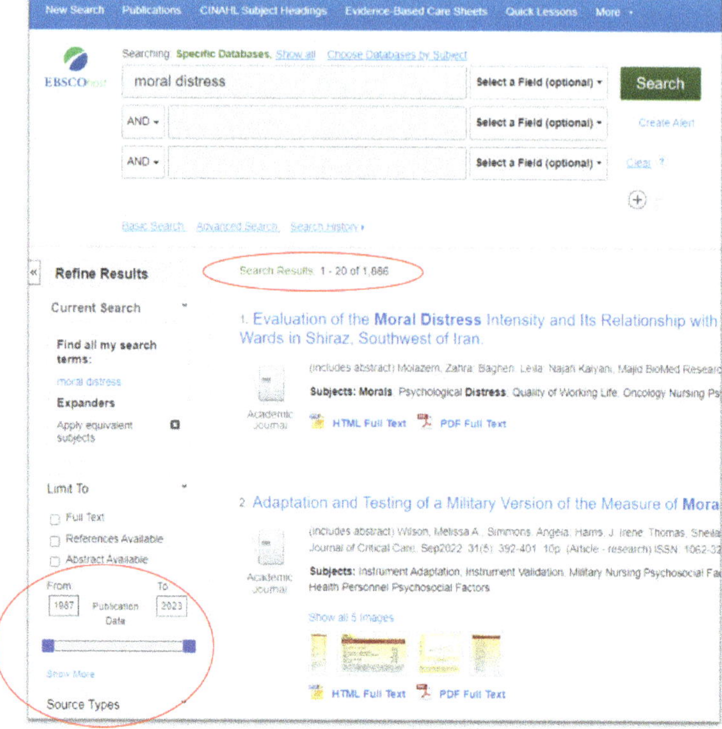

FIGURE 7.2 Search for the word phrase "moral distress," which returned 1,886 results with a time span of 1987–2023

The second image shows the dialog box for the subject major headings filter.

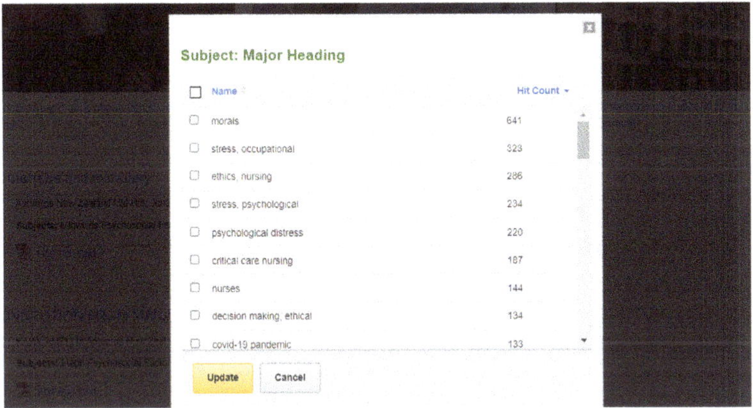

FIGURE 7.3 Image of the dialog box that opens to show the exact count of results tied to subtopics within the subject major heading filter.

Notice the hit count numbers on the right side of the dialog box for each subject major heading. Tick boxes are on the left side of the dialog box. If the choices are clear, researchers can select one or more tick boxes to narrow the results in an informed way. Also, researchers might want to examine the results of each sub-topic one by one. This system permits careful study of the contents found within the 1,886 results. The Subject Major headings filter provides a useful way to explore and choose a subset of articles from total search results. This analysis helps researchers include or exclude articles in an exact way. Researchers might develop their inclusion and exclusion criteria more easily by analyzing these data.

Another tip is that CINAHL searches groups of terms from left to right. After searching the first set of terms on the left, CINAHL returns results on the left set of terms first. Next CINAHL searches within the second set of terms. This feature means that how the search terms are ordered in the search screens affects how CINAHL conducts the search.

Another feature for CINAHL and similar EBSCOhost databases is that multiple filters are available. Researchers might use the table below (see Table 7.1) to record search decisions and results. This table is valuable for the Search Strategy figure in the PowerPoint slide presentation. Researchers would transfer data from this table

TABLE 7.1 Table to be Used to Record Searches, Search Decisions, and Results

CINAHL	Date/time		# hits	Time span	Decision
Key words	Close cousin words	Boolean Operators			
Moral distress	None used	None	1,886	1987-2023	Check subject major headings

to the PowerPoint Search Strategy figure to show the researcher's path to the final set of articles.

Use Boolean Operators Properly

Most library databases use three specific Boolean operator commands to help the database select and compile articles. Three Boolean operator words are: AND, OR, and NOT. Boolean operators are typically written into search sentences with ALL CAPS to differentiate them from search terms. Keep in mind that Boolean operators are not acronyms. It is important to know that each database provides its own Boolean operators. In CINAHL, they sit between the search lines on a search screen like a stairway from one floor to the next. In PubMed, the software builds Boolean operators into a search sentence when conducting an advanced search. However, Boolean operators are not search terms, so they may not be put into search screens or search lines by researchers. They must be used according to the software program's own rules.

The Boolean operator AND tells a search engine to narrow the search by joining all words within the parenthetical phrase with each other. This means that if I put two search terms into two lines of a search screen, such as neonate in the top line and teen parent in the second line, the default Boolean operator AND would tell the database to search for articles that include the word 'neonate' and the phrase 'teen parent.' In CINAHL, AND is the default Boolean operator.

In contrast, the Boolean operator/command OR tells the search engine to explode or broaden the search by looking for articles with any words joined by OR within the parenthetical phrase. That means that if I put the two search terms above and used the Boolean operator OR, the database would search separately for 'neonate' and for 'teen parents.' See below.

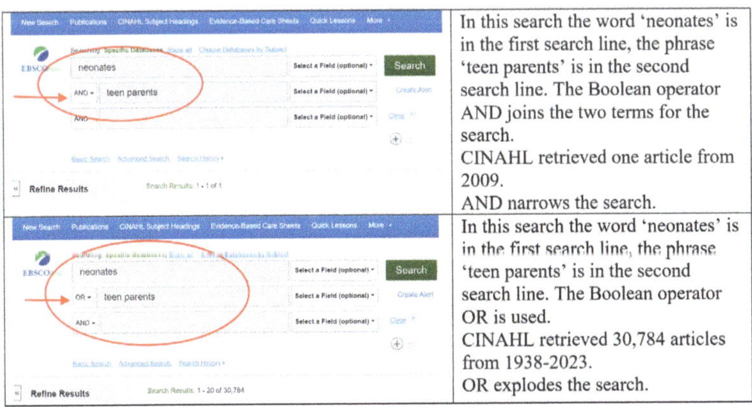

AND search	In this search the word 'neonates' is in the first search line, the phrase 'teen parents' is in the second search line. The Boolean operator AND joins the two terms for the search. CINAHL retrieved one article from 2009. AND narrows the search.
OR search	In this search the word 'neonates' is in the first search line, the phrase 'teen parents' is in the second search line. The Boolean operator OR is used. CINAHL retrieved 30,784 articles from 1938-2023. OR explodes the search.

FIGURE 7.4 Examples of Boolean operators. AND is in the top box. OR is in the lower box.

The first example shows the Boolean operator AND, which joined two search terms to narrow a search. One article from 2009 was retrieved. The second example shows the Boolean operator OR. The articles found contain either the term neonates OR the phrase teen parents.

Finally, the Boolean operator NOT tells the search engine to exclude articles with the NOT term from the prior search. In the third search below, the same terms, 'neonates' and 'teen parents' were used with Boolean operator OR. A search term was added on a third search line to exclude articles about animals. The Boolean operator NOT was added with the search term 'animal.' This reduced results by three articles to 30,781. The time frame was the same, 1938-2023.

The third Boolean connector, NOT, excludes any articles with the NOT word. For example (neonates, infants, newborns, babies) AND (human) NOT (animal). This set of search commands tells the search engine to retrieve articles that are about either human neonates or infants or newborns or babies, and to exclude any research about baby animals or newborn or neonate or infant animals. Using NOT is useful if your major search terms could be for populations other than human beings, such as NOT animal, or NOT robotic or NOT virtual or NOT simulated.

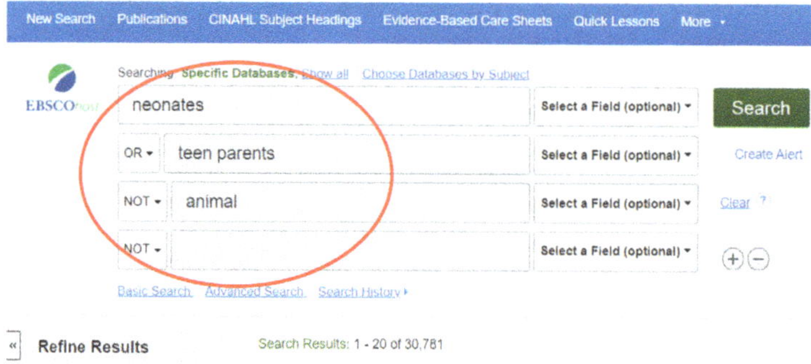

FIGURE 7.5 Screenshot of CINAHL search with OR and NOT Boolean operators

To recap: An incorrect or misplaced use of Boolean operators, such as OR instead of AND can play havoc with a search. The Boolean operator AND joins words to make searches more specific. The Boolean operator OR explodes a search. In 1999 when I searched for articles about moral distress, I used the phrase: "moral" AND "distress" to indicate that the words "moral" and "distress" must always be present in the articles. However, when I examined the articles provided from that search, I realized it was not an accurate search. Then I learned that I should write the search command as "moral distress." Quotation marks around the word phrase would tell CINAHL to keep the two search words, moral and distress together in that exact order. That approach was useful.

In contrast, the Boolean operator OR broadens searches by searching for and retrieving articles with all the words. If I had put the terms "moral" OR "distress" I would have received more articles that contained either word, but little relevant evidence about the topic of 'moral distress' itself. Of note, all 'or' words written in lowercase letters are not Boolean operators. When researchers put a group of close cousin words together, such as (neonate or infant or newborn or baby), that lower case 'or' between the close cousin words does not act as a Boolean operator. Remember that CINAHL searches for words from left to right within word phrases. Boolean operators join or separate terms from search line to search line.

Incorrect Use of Boolean Operators

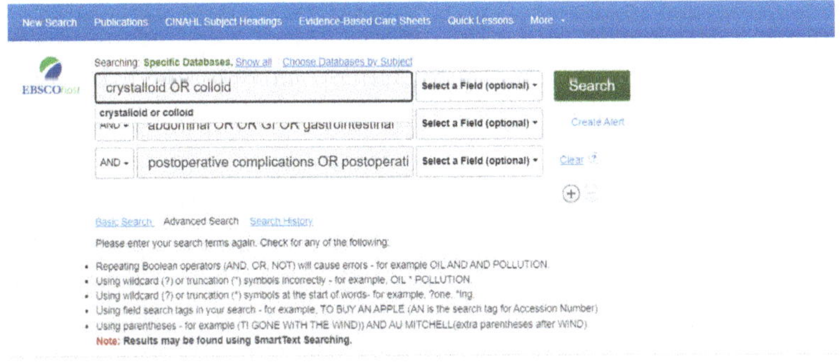

FIGURE 7.6 Screenshot of CINAHL'S warning about using ALL CAPS within a phrase.

Notice that the terms "crystalloid OR colloid" in the first search line prompt CINAHL to offer a drop down menu with the proper combination of search terms. Underneath the search lines, CINAHL requests users to enter the search terms again. CINAHL also brings up a warning that repeating Boolean operators will cause errors. That also prompted CINAHL to give more information and directions about how to search. In fact, the notes mention wild cards and truncation.

Wild Card Commands

Another type of command that databases recognize is a form of special punctuation called 'wild card' characters. Four common wild card characters are *, ?, $, and #. The exact wild card character can differ from one database to another. Wildcard characters can be inserted into, in front of or at the end of a search term. For example, researchers want articles written in English. They are aware that their search term has two different spellings: an American English spelling, such as color, and a British English spelling, such as colour. Researchers can insert the wild card character # in the American spelling (colo#r) to retrieve articles with either spelling. Another popular wild card character is the asterisk, *. Researchers can place an asterisk at the end of a word stem, such as nurs* to truncate a term and then retrieve all the variations of that term. This use of the asterisk wild card with the word stem 'nurs*' would bring up articles with the terms nurse, nurses, nursing, and nursology. Readers would help themselves by reviewing each library database's FAQs or tutorials before using an unfamiliar database.

In healthcare related databases such as CINAHL or PubMed, age is another useful filter category. For example, an investigator using CINAHL can limit articles to those that mention age such as adults, geriatrics, or pediatrics. Finally, the limit that is often misused and improperly timed is the limit for publication years. If this limit is placed too early in the search, or if it is used as the first choice to reduce the results, researchers will lose a chance to analyze the full body of evidence about their topic. In fact, they won't have any idea how large the true body of evidence is. Information about the chronological time of publication is a great gift of knowledge. It should be used well, not discarded too quickly.

Certain databases indicate the date range for all publications with each search. For example, if the term "music therapy" is put into the CINAHL database, a dropdown screen shows alternative words: music therapy or music intervention or musical therapy. When clicking on that set of terms, the database returns 9,716 articles that would meet the search terms. At the same time, CINAHL shows the range of publication years for all the articles: 1957-2023.

Evidence-based researchers who work in a strict manner could cut off all articles earlier than 2017. To do this in CINAHL, users would change 1957 to 2017 and hit 'enter' again. By snipping off six decades of publications, without having examined the body of evidence during those sixty years, the total number of articles was reduced to 3,348. At the same time, 6,368 articles were removed from consideration. Without having checked any other filters, researchers lost the chance to learn where the articles originated (geography), age of populations where music therapy was used, or which topics were of interest over time (subject major headings).

So far in this chapter, only the P portion of the search sentence has been set up. Yet, PICO questions have about four, sometimes five sets of major search terms. When a PICO/T question is written, where T stands for Time, that kind of major search term about time is different from the 'publication year' limit. What each filter and limit means, and how they are used will be discussed below as the search process is presented in detail.

Translating Search Strategies into Search Sentences

Search strategies use five types of database commands to retrieve evidence. Five commands are 1) Major search terms or a controlled vocabulary, 2) Filters, 3) Limits, 4) Boolean operators, and 5) Wild Cards. Major search terms are the first commands needed for useful search sentences. These are the P-I-C-O and close cousin words. When telling the evidence story, researchers summarize the search strategy by writing a search sentence. For example, to write the first part of a search sentence with the P word, neonate, including three close cousin words, the sentence might look like: In (neonat* or infant* or newborn* or baby) … The asterisk helps to truncate the term neonate so that the database will also search for the words neonatal and neonates. The words 'infant' and 'newborn' are truncated with an asterisk so that the database search will include infant, infants, newborn, newborns.

This first part of the search sentence lists the P word first followed by three close cousin words. To write the search sentence, the P word phrase is separated from other phrases in the sentence with parentheses. Parentheses around search phrases are a command that certain databases recognize and use. For example, when using the advanced search feature in PubMed, each choice is built into a search sentence. PubMed puts parentheses around search term groups. The parentheses tell the database to search for those four words in the order they appear in the group. The database will search for the first word, then for the second word, then for the third word and last, the fourth word.

Phrases link together to become full search sentences. The true function of search sentences is to show the full set of commands given to library databases to find relevant evidence. The search sentence is the final record of commands given to databases to find the evidence. A good search sentence is written last so that future researchers will be able to verify and replicate that study.

One difference between CINAHL and PubMed, is that CINAHL uses the subject major heading filter. CINAHL offers drop down menu suggestions based on subject major headings, which are usually excellent close cousin terms. PubMed can show MeSH terms (Medical Subject Headings) from a menu, but it does not automatically populate the search lines with possible terms. Also, in PubMed Boolean operators appear while a search sentence is being built in the advanced search screen. In both databases, Boolean operators are within the database software. They cannot be imposed as a search term in the search screens.

Structure of Search Sentences

Search sentences show the full set of results of interactive analytical search efforts. They are placed into the top box of the PowerPoint Search Strategy figure in the evidence-based research presentation. The search sentence is composed of parenthetical phrases that each contain the P-I-C-O search terms, Boolean operators that connect each phrase, and last with limits and filters added underneath the search sentence as additional information. The purpose of placing the full search sentence into the final presentation is so that viewers will be able to evaluate the adequacy of the search used to compile the evidence set. Also, if the evidence-based project is presented externally, the full search sentence would help others replicate the search.

CINAHL does not accept a formal, complete search sentence as a search term. PubMed permits researchers to create a full search sentence in the Advanced Search area. When a complete search sentence is entered into a library database, the results should be the most relevant articles needed to answer the original PICO question. What makes search sentences effective? Search sentences are effective when they use the best major search terms [major subject headings or MeSH headings], correct Boolean operators, proper punctuation, and the preferred format for that electronic database.

Prudent Approaches to Choosing Search Terms

The choices people make when searching in a library database affect the relevance and quality of published articles found during the search. Remember when the 'P' word was neonates? The investigator needed to choose close cousin words to develop an efficient search sentence. A quick look at a thesaurus page from *dictionary.com website* brought up a variety of synonyms for the word 'neonate' that most scientific researchers would never use. Scientists use scientific words that are precise, accurate and objective. Words like toddler, child and kid apply to children older than neonates, so those words are not accurate. Words like babe, cherub, and darling are slang terms that are not objective, scholarly words, so they would not be used either. From the two examinations of words, four words are reasonable alternative words in the search sentence: neonate, infant, newborn, and baby. Once the set of exact search words is known the next decision is which Boolean operator should connect those four words in the P part of the search sentence?

As each part of the search sentence is developed into separate parenthetical phrases with the precise PICO words, all close cousins, correct Boolean operators, and the parentheses, the entire sentence is completed by putting all the parenthetical phrases into a single sentence. The complete search sentence is placed into the top box of the PowerPoint Search Figure slide for the final presentation.

This part of the search strategy figure shows the path taken to identify evidence.

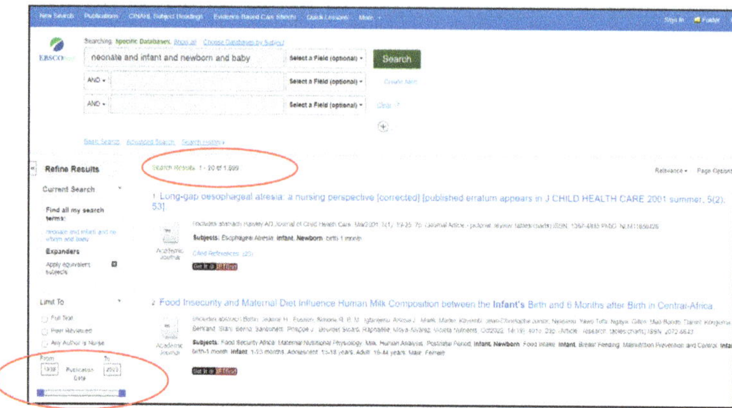

FIGURE 7.7 Screenshot of CINAHL search with neonate and infant and newborn and baby retrieves 1,699 records from 1938–2023.

If a researcher used the lower case word 'or,' that word would make each word separate from the others. The command to the database would be to search for any of the terms in that phrase.

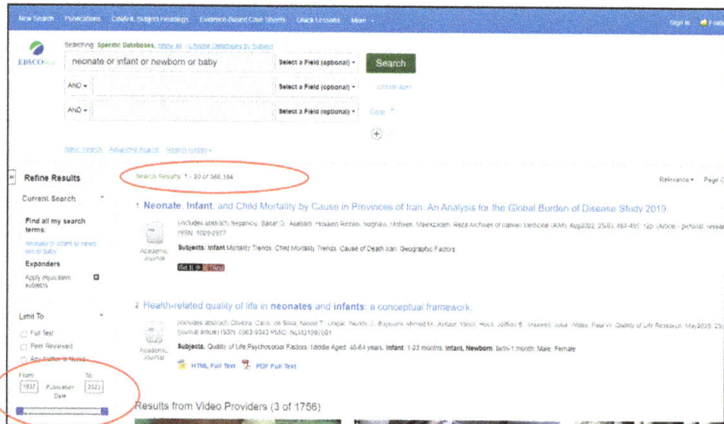

FIGURE 7.8 Screenshot of CINAHL search for neonate or infant or newborn or baby which shows 358,184 records. The years for all those records are from 1937–2023.

The ALL CAPS '**AND,**' is a Boolean operator. It connects two levels of words like a staircase connects two floors in a building. **OR** and **NOT** are recognized by the database as Boolean operator commands. When lowercase letters are used, and the words 'and' 'or' or 'not' are placed within parentheses as part of a search phrase, CINAHL will use all the words in that phrase as instructed. When two major search terms are linked with 'and,' CINAHL will only look for articles that include both words. For example, if the evidence-based researcher put two major search terms into a search line, (moral and distress), CINAHL would search for all articles that contain the two words in the order given: moral, distress. First, CINAHL would search for all articles that have the word moral. Next, CINAHL would search for all articles that have the word distress. However, if an evidence-based researcher wanted evidence on the topic of "moral distress" CINAHL would search only for articles that have those two major search terms in exactly that order with quotation marks.

Searching in PubMed.gov

PubMed.gov is a free, United States government-sponsored electronic database available through the U. S. National Library of Medicine website. This database is dedicated to biomedical information, so it serves the interests of physicians and biomedical scientists very well. PubMed is much larger than CINAHL, with approximately 35,000,000 articles compared with CINHAL's approximately 4,000,000 articles. PubMed is continuously updating its capability. It has a new feature called 'proximity searching.' This is a search feature that differs from how the CINAHL database searches for records. Recall that CINAHL searches for the terms in the order they are listed from left to right. With proximity searching PubMed searches for multiple terms in any order within a specified distance of each other. For example, PubMed could search for terms in titles and abstracts simultaneously.

PubMed features are like CINAHL's, but they are also unique. Even though PubMed has the same filters as CINAHL, when PubMed's filters are opened the chance to specify and narrow the filter is greater in PubMed than in CINAHL. For example, CINAHL's age filter breaks into general categories: pediatric, adolescent, adult, and older adult. PubMed uses narrow, specific age ranges. PubMed also provides a graphic chart with the timeline for all articles retrieved. Since the PubMed database is nine times larger than CINAHL's, PubMed typically returns more results. See Figure 7.9 below, a screenshot of PubMed's results for the same word phrase previously put into CINAHL: moral distress.

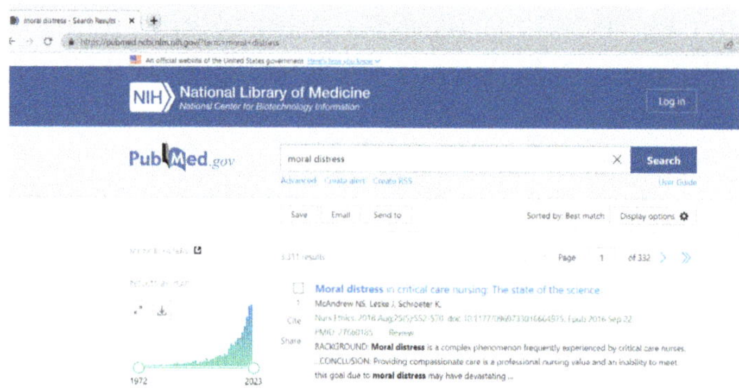

FIGURE 7.9 Image of PubMed search results for the word phrase 'moral distress'

Recall that in CINAHL the word phrase, 'moral distress,' brought up 1,886 results with a timeline from 1987-2023. In PubMed, the phrase 'moral distress' brought up 3,311 results with a timeline from 1972-2023. Even though the top citation in PubMed is related to nursing, the article is from 2018. The top citation in CINAHL, which is dedicated to nursing and allied health journals, is from 2022.

The comparison shows that it is worthwhile to search at least two databases when conducting an evidence-based research project. There will often be a degree of overlap between the two searches, but there will also be unique results.

Final Words About Two Search Skills: How to Search, How to Filter Searches

In this chapter two skills were presented together since the work and tasks for these skills overlap with each other. To learn how to search in electronic databases, it is important to start learning about what each database offers, how it operates, and if it has any unique features. It is also important to learn the limits of each database. Limits do exist. Library databases, unlike internet search engines, are usually more reliable in terms of the quality of results they provide. There is less chance that fake or predatory journal articles will be found in library databases. The library database owners are careful about which journal articles, or conference abstracts may be included. Each database has tutorial information. It is possible to learn how to search in the main databases of one's discipline. It is important to keep track of all search efforts and decisions for each search strategy. The data is embedded in the Search Figure for the final presentation of research findings. A clear and well-documented search strategy is a sign of high-quality work.

References

EBSCOhost. https://www.ebsco.com/products/ebscohost-research-platform

ProQuest. https://about.proquest.com/en/about/who-we-are/

WoltersKluwer. https://www.wolterskluwer.com/en/solutions/ovid/platforms-products/databases

Credits

Figures 7.1–7.8: Generated with CINAHL Database. Copyright © by EBSCO Information Services.

Fig. 7.9: Generated with PubMed, https://pubmed.ncbi.nlm.nih.gov/. National Library of Medicine, U.S. Department of Health and Human Services (HHS).

CHAPTER 8

Skill 4

Create Evidence Table Shells

LEARNING GOALS

1. Create two basic table shells to display distinct types of evidence.
2. Extract relevant data and add it to evidence tables.
3. Use meaningful icons to show the evidence story in the final synthesis tables.

The Purpose of Evidence Tables

Researchers use evidence tables to sift the evidence and sort relevant data to tell the evidence story in a clear, logical way. One type of table shows **critical appraisal reviews** of each article. Another type, **evidence display tables**, shows how certain variables, such as interventions, patient characteristics, outcomes, adverse events, costs, benefits, social determinants of health, or other data, cluster together. Three other tables show 1) type and quality of evidence, 2) full evidence summary, and 3) synthesis of findings for the entire **evidence set**. The evidence set refers to the entire group of articles kept after the screening of articles ends.

Before creating basic table shells, researchers must put their entire evidence set in order. They must number each evidence item, preferably in a two-digit format. Researchers use a variety of ways to order their evidence. In this guide, I advise readers to arrange evidence in historical order. Put the oldest articles first and the newest publications last. The effect of historical order is that researchers will be able to show how evidence has evolved over time. This approach is meaningful especially if the evidence shows a conceptual or theoretical "break." For example, the COVID-19 pandemic gave health professionals a conceptual break related to how to treat severe hypoxia. Prior to COVID-19, respiratory technology and algorithms to treat severe hypoxia were complex and powerful. During COVID-19, the algorithms and technology failed repeatedly. The conceptual break with our former way of thinking came in April 2020. Our Italian colleagues in Lombardy, Italy reported success with a low-tech treatment, prone positioning, in the open access journal JAMA Network (Grasselli et al., 2020).

This low-tech treatment held a glimmer of hope for patient survival. Readers might recall that in April 2020, no medications or vaccines were yet available. Before COVID-19, patients with severe hypoxia were treated with intubation, mechanical ventilation, high levels of inspired oxygen, and high positive end-expiratory pressure (PEEP) to push oxygen into the pulmonary system. If that failed, patients might receive an even higher-tech treatment called ECMO (extra-corporeal membrane oxygenation). During COVID, even ECMO failed certain patients. Italian physicians went for broke when they turned toward prone positioning. That low-tech treatment was previously used for a condition called acute respiratory distress syndrome (ARDS). One key symptom of ARDS is pink, frothy sputum. Although COVID patients did not have that symptom, like patients with ARDS, they had severe hypoxia unresponsive to other treatments. Once patients were positioned on their abdomens, they were finally able to breathe. That April 2020 idea of treating COVID-19 with low-tech prone positioning was a conceptual break idea during the early pandemic.

If researchers disregard the evidence story's history, they might lose a key before/after aspect of it. For this book, I ask readers to arrange their articles in historical order, with oldest publications first and newest last. A conceptual break in ideas might be revealed.

When evidence tables are complete, researchers analyze them to understand the body of evidence. Based on that analysis, researchers advise evidence-based changes if needed. When evidence tables are clear, they logically reveal a compelling evidence story to stakeholders during the presentation of final findings.

Develop Basic Table Shells

Researchers start with two basic **table shells**. One table, called the **evidence display table**, shows the evidence from all articles for each category of evidence. The other table, called a **critical appraisal table**, shows evidence from each article. The evidence display table shell shows distinct types of data from the evidence set (see Table 8.1 below). It has one wide empty first column followed by narrow columns. When the table shell is created, researchers must put enough columns to display data from each article in the definitive evidence set. The display table shell has article numbers in the top horizontal line in a two-digit format. Beneath the table is a key of brief references numbered to correspond with column numbers. A finished basic display table shell for nine articles is shown in Table 8.1. When evidence sets have 10 or more pieces of evidence, the 10th reference can be automatically reordered by some word processing programs to be next the single-digit number one. The reason to use a two-digit format is to ensure the numbers and brief references in the key will stay in order.

TABLE 8.1 Basic Evidence Display Table Shell

List the evidence category here	01	02	03	04	05	06	07	08	09

Key: *01 Author, xxxx; 02 Author, xxxx; 03 Author, xxxx; 04 Author, xxxx; 05 Author, xxxx; 06 Author, xxxx; 07 Author, xxxx; 08 Author, xxxx; 09 Author, xxxx.*

For instructions on how to set up a basic evidence display table shell, see Appendix A. Once a table shell is set up, duplicate the display table shell at least 10 times. The tables will display separate types of data. For example, tables can display the variety of interventions, comparison interventions, benefits, costs, adverse events, social determinants of health, positive and negative outcomes, and other elements found in the data. Display tables show the frequency of separate categories of evidence extracted from each report.

Stakeholders will follow an evidence story more easily during the presentation if evidence display tables have a uniform underlying structure.

Critical Appraisal Table Shell

Critical appraisal of evidence is at the heart of evidence-based practice. The **Critical Appraisal table shell** conveys specific data extracted from each article. In this chapter, an author-generated critical appraisal table shell is presented and discussed (see Table 8.2 below, and Appendix B).

Critical appraisal is a thorough review of each piece of evidence based on standards for that type of evidence. For example, a thorough review of a randomized controlled trial will focus on distinct aspects of an experimental study. A review of a mailed survey will focus on details like the response rate and sampling frame. In the critical appraisal table shell, researchers can record key elements of each piece of evidence. It is important to put the article's number, which will appear on all evidence display tables, and the full reference at the top of the table. Underneath the first row of information is a series of six columns. Column 1 is for the category and type of evidence. In this table, numbers for the type of evidence come from the research and nonresearch figures shown in Chapter 9. However, researchers are free to build their critical appraisal with levels of evidence from other evidence-based practice texts. If using the Johns Hopkins Evidence-Based Practice textbook, there are five levels of evidence. If using the text by Melnyk and Fineout-Overholt, there are seven levels of evidence. If using the text by Polit and Beck, there are eight levels of evidence. It is important to use the

TABLE 8.2 Critical Appraisal Table Shell

<table>
<tr><td>01</td><td colspan="6">Author Name(s). (year). Article title. Journal Title, vol.# (issue #), page numbers.</td></tr>
<tr><td colspan="2">Category & Level of evidence
Research 1, 2, 3, 4
Non-Research 5, 6, 7, 8</td><td>Method
Quant
Experimental
Quasi-experimental
Non-experimental
Qual
Phenomenology
Grounded Theory
Ethnography

Mixed Methods</td><td>Sample Population

Sample size
N = ___

Type of sample</td><td>Variables Concepts

Interventions (IV)

Outcomes (DV)

Themes</td><td>Data collection

Analysis

Instruments</td><td>Findings

Strengths

Limitations

Interpretation</td></tr>
<tr><td colspan="3">Author credentials</td><td colspan="3">Reviewer's comments:</td><td>Quality of evidence</td></tr>
</table>

evidence-based practice model that fits with the reader's current institutional model. Column 2 lists the possible methods from large categories of quantitative, qualitative, mixed methods, and subsets underneath those methods. When completing this column, simply remove the elements that do not apply to simplify the table. In column 3, researchers have room to put information about the sampling plan. For nonresearch articles, a sampling plan does not apply. For quantitative studies, it is important to know of sample characteristics such as a random or nonrandom sample, sample size (N = XX), and any relevant aspects to describe the sample.

Column 4 is the variables column. Researchers can list interventions (also called independent variables), outcomes (also called the dependent variables), and any themes, patterns, or concepts noted. Column 4 information is used to develop a variety of evidence display tables. Column 4 is a good place to put notes about adverse events, benefits, or costs.

In Column 5, researchers put the data collection, management, and analysis plan. If any instruments were used to collect data, that information should go in column 5. Any statistical results would be put into column 5. This leaves column 6 for a concise report of findings, study strengths and limitations, and relevant comments about interpretation of data.

In the next row, which is divided into three separate boxes, researchers can put information about the authors' credentials, a larger box for summary comments about the study, and a last box for researchers to determine whether the evidence is high quality, medium quality, or low quality. How to evaluate the quality of evidence is presented in Chapter 10.

As researchers review each piece of evidence, they will extract data bits from each article and transfer those data bits to display tables. An example of a research critical appraisal table shell is in Appendix B.

Presenting the Evidence Story to Stakeholders

When presenting the evidence story to stakeholders, researchers copy each critical appraisal table onto blank slides of a Microsoft PowerPoint presentation. Researchers can create their critical appraisal table shell on an 11" x 17" blank Microsoft Word document in landscape layout. A spacious layout helps researchers when typing essential elements into the table for the first time. In contrast, a PP slide is much smaller than an 11" x 17" document. The content would be reduced to barely readable font if each table were copied and pasted directly onto a PP slide. To make each critical appraisal table fit onto blank PowerPoint slides, it is best to work first with a large document. Next, edit the table for conciseness. Finally, copy the reduced table onto a blank PowerPoint slide. This chapter gives chances to build separate evidence tables.

Classifying Evidence: Types or Levels

Readers of this book will classify evidence by type. Other evidence-based practice books classify evidence according to levels based on a pyramid structure. This book does not use a pyramid. For learning purposes, this book uses two rectangular figures that show four types of research evidence and four kinds of nonresearch evidence (see Chapter 9, Figures 9.1 and 9.2). Depending on the evidence-based practice model that a reader must use for an employer's selected model of evidence-based practice, the types or levels of evidence can be as few as five (such as with the Johns Hopkins Evidence-Based Practice Model), or seven (such as with the Melnyk/Fineout-Overholt EBP model) or eight (such as with the Polit/Beck EBP research model). Researchers must indicate the EBP model in use when presenting the evidence story. Use one evidence display table to show the types or levels of evidence for the entire evidence set according to that model. The types or levels of evidence table helps stakeholders grasp the shape of the body of evidence during the final presentation. To keep things simple for this chapter, Table 8.3 shows eight types of evidence.

The types of evidence table is set up with the evidence display table shell.

Variables and Evidence Display Tables

Evidence display tables are designed to show which articles have different pieces of evidence. Data extracted from the evidence are often called variables. Quantitative research usually has three types of variables: independent variables, dependent variables, and confounding or extraneous variables. Group each type of variable into a table with similar variables. For example, put intervention variables, also called independent variables, into intervention tables. Depending on the evidence being explored, researchers might find they have subtopics within each variable type. Some interventions might be active; other interventions might be passive in nature. Another category of evidence display table shows the effects or outcomes of the interventions. Effects or outcomes are also called dependent variables. It is possible to find a third category of variables

TABLE 8.3 Types of Evidence Column Shows What Constitutes Each Type of Evidence with an Assigned Number

Types of Evidence	01	02	03	04	05	06	07	08
Type 1 [RCTs/experimental]								
Type 2 [quasi-experimental]								
Type 3 [non-experimental]								
Type 4 [multiple research]								
Type 5 [nonresearch: consensus]								
Type 6 [nonresearch: clinical guidelines]								
Type 7 [nonresearch: case study]								
Type 8 [nonresearch: expert opinion, editorial]								

Key: *01 Green, 2019; 02 Brown, 2019; 03 Gold, 2020; 04 McKenna, 2020; 05 Justin, 2021; 06 Saverio, 2022; 07 Celeste, 2022; 08 Olson, 2023.*

Number remaining columns at the top in two-digit format to match the articles listed in the key beneath the table. The key shows the first author's last name and publication year for each piece of evidence.

called extraneous or confounding variables in the evidence. These variables are not part of the research design, but they can negatively affect final findings. Rarely, researchers have serendipitous findings, which are positive unanticipated findings.

Each broad category of variables has subcategories, such as active interventions, passive interventions, positive outcomes, negative outcomes, costs, and benefits. To assemble display tables, sort data into categories. Display data by categories using separate display tables. Stakeholders will follow a story that is logical and clear.

Experimental and quasi-experimental studies usually have an **intervention**, which is also called a "manipulation." Interventions given to experimental groups and withheld from control groups are experimental interventions. Experimental interventions are

TABLE 8.4 Interventions Display Table with Potential Subcategories Listed

Interventions Display Table	01	02	03	04	05	06	07	08	09
Active interventions									
Passive interventions									
Combined interventions									
Thwarted interventions									

Key: 01 Green, 2019; 02 Brown, 2019; 03 Gold, 2020; 04 McKenna, 2020; 05 Justin, 2021; 06 Saverio, 2022; 07 Celeste, 2022; 08 Olson, 2023; 09 Lennon, 2023.

independent variables. Effects or outcomes of interventions are **dependent variables.** When evidence-based researchers gather evidence about a single topic, it is possible that studies can have a variety of independent variables (a variety of interventions) to answer questions about the same topic.

Different Uses for Evidence Display Tables

For an interventions display table, list all the interventions from the body of evidence in the first column. In the numbered columns, place an X to show which articles mention the interventions. Complete one vertical column for each piece of evidence. If there is no information about an intervention in an article, leave that box blank. Column numbers at the top of the table must match the key below. Use table shells to display evidence in historical order. Keeping that order during the researcher's work maximizes understanding of how the evidence evolved over time.

A body of research evidence to answer a specific PICO question can have distinct types of interventions (independent variables). Likewise, the evidence can contain a variety of outcomes (dependent variables). Besides the independent and dependent variables, research evidence that mentions extraneous or confounding variables might provide insight into the body of evidence. All ideas are important when considering the complete body of evidence to answer a specific PICO question.

Experienced evidence-based researchers create multiple evidence tables from the basic table shell before engaging in critical appraisal. Setting up table shells after the first comprehensive reading of evidence, and again after adjustments to the final evidence set are complete, makes critical appraisal more efficient.

Outcomes of Evidence Display Tables

The body of evidence can reveal a variety of effects, also called outcomes or dependent variables. Notice in the table below that the qualities of dependent variables can be positive or negative, desirable or undesirable, expected or unexpected, or a true surprise, serendipitous. The display tables show stakeholders all ideas found in the evidence.

TABLE 8.5 Outcomes of Evidence Display Table

Outcomes Display Table	01	02	03	04	05	06	07	08	09
Positive or desirable outcomes									
Negative or undesirable outcomes									
Expected outcomes									
Unexpected outcomes									
Serendipitous outcomes									

Key: 01 Green, 2019; 02 Brown, 2019; 03 Gold, 2020; 04 McKenna, 2020; 05 Justin, 2021; 06 Saverio, 2022; 07 Celeste, 2022; 08 Olson, 2023; 09 Lennon, 2023.

Social Determinants of Health and/or Diversity, Equity, Inclusion Display Tables

Another form of intervention and/or outcome that is often not shown in the evidence is based on social determinants of health. When researchers understand how social determinants of health can silently affect the evidence, it becomes a moral-ethical matter to seek data about those determinants. For example, if a quantitative study reports demographic data for a patient population, such as age and gender, but fails to mention whether people in the study were impoverished, homeless, or uneducated, how will researchers be able to effectively evaluate that evidence? To tell a valid story, evidence must not silently exclude any factor that might influence the story. In this book, evidence display tables can be used to show missing data about the social determinants of health.

To recap: Consideration of social determinants of health is often a missing piece of evidence-based research. It is time to include that level of analysis during critical appraisal. Create separate evidence display tables to show relevant aspects of social determinants of health (see Table 8.6 below). Castrucci and Auerbach's (2019) theory

TABLE 8.6 Social Determinants of Health Evidence Display Table

SDOH Display Table	01	02	03	04	05	06	07	08	09
Economic stability factors									
Education factors									
Social and community context factors									
Health and health care factors									
Neighborhood & built environment factors									

Key: *01 Green, 2019; 02 Brown, 2019; 03 Gold, 2020; 04 McKenna, 2020; 05 Justin, 2021; 06 Saverio, 2022; 07 Celeste, 2022; 08 Olson, 2023; 09 Lennon, 2023.*

(Based on Castrucci & Auerbach, 2019)

of social determinants of health can inform such a display table. Chapter Two of *The Future of Nursing 2020–2030: Charting a Path to Achieve Health Equity* (2021) describes Castrucci and Auerbach's theory of social determinants of health in detail. A brief synopsis of that theory is below.

Social determinants of health include five major areas: 1) economic stability, 2) education, 3) social and community context, 4) health and health care, and 5) neighborhood and built environment. Each major area contains several subtopics. For example, the area of economic stability includes subtopics of employment, food insecurity, housing instability, and poverty. How would an evidence-based researcher use the employment subtopic during critical appraisal? A question about the subtopic of employment might be, does the demographic data include a category such as employed full-time, employed part-time, occasionally employed, unemployed, or is the topic of employment not mentioned at all? Evidence display tables show the evidence present in each article. If social determinants of health categories are not present, it might be necessary to create tables that reveal the presence and absence of specific determinants.

Synthesis Tables

Synthesized evidence requires a distinct look. Rather than Xs, the synthesis table uses meaningful icons to represent the synthesis of evidence. Whereas the interventions and outcomes tables show where the evidence was located among the research reports, the synthesis table is designed to tell the story of what the interventions and their outcomes mean. This is where evidence-based researchers use meaningful icons to display the evidence so that the advice that follows will be logically connected to the evidence.

Notice that for each synthesized outcome, an icon and color are used to depict the meaning. Common colors to use in synthesis tables are red, yellow, and green, the stoplight colors. Green is often used for outcomes that are desirable. Green lights mean go. Red lights mean stop. Red icons are used to show an undesirable or negative outcome. Yellow is a stoplight's "slow down" or "caution"

TABLE 8.7 Evidence Synthesis Table

Evidence Synthesis Table	01	02	03	04	05	06	07	08	09
Positive or desirable outcomes	↑								
Negative or undesirable outcomes		↓							
Expected outcomes—Good			♥						
Unexpected outcomes—Not Good				⚡					
Serendipitous outcomes—Good					☺				

Key: 01 Green, 2019; 02 Brown, 2019; Gold, 2020; 04 McKenna, 2020; 05 Justin, 2021; 06 Saverio, 2022; 07 Celeste, 2022; 08 Olson, 2023; 09 Lennon, 2023.

color. Icons in yellow could signify a “slow down” or “be careful” meaning. The other colors, such as purple for a lightning bolt and a blue outlined happy face, are arbitrary colors selected to contrast the other colors. By the time stakeholders view the synthesis table, they will have already seen the display tables, where the evidence is concentrated. The synthesis of evidence should confirm stakeholders’ understanding of the evidence story as it was told.

After the evidence synthesis is conveyed, researchers come to the final pieces of advice for future action. They will either outline a plan to translate the new evidence into work-related changes, or they will affirm that no changes are needed at present. If the advice is for novel changes, having an outline of those changes will engage stakeholders in mutual, collaborative problem-solving to achieve those new goals.

References

Castrucci B. C., Auerbach J. (2019, January 19). Meeting individual social needs falls short of addressing social determinants of health. HealthAffairs. https://www.healthaffairs.org/do/10.1377/hblog20190115.234942/full/

Grasselli, G., Zangrillo, A., Zanella, A., Antonelli, M., Cabrini, L., Castelli, A., Cereda, D., Coluccello, A., Foti, G., Fumagalli, R., Iotti, G., Latronico, N., Lorini, L., Merler, S., Natalini, G., Piatti, A., Ranieri, M. V., Scandroglio, A.M., Storti, E., … COVID-19 Lombardy ICU Network. (2020). Baseline characteristics and outcomes of 1591 patients infected with SARS-CoV-2 admitted to the ICUs of Lombardy Region Italy. *JAMA Network, 323*(16), 1574–1581.

National Academies of Sciences, Engineering, and Medicine. (2021). *The future of nursing 2020–2030: Charting a path to achieve health equity.* National Academies Press. https://doi.org/10.17226/25982

Credits

ICN 8.1: Copyright © 2020 Depositphotos/Mandarin007.
ICN 8.2: Copyright © 2020 Depositphotos/Mandarin007.
ICN 8.3: Copyright © 2019 Depositphotos/Tornadodesign.
ICN 8.4: Copyright © 2020 Depositphotos/Monory.
ICN 8.5: Copyright © 2019 Depositphotos/rootstocks.

CHAPTER 9

Skill 5

Critical Appraisal, Part I

LEARNING GOALS

1. Explain four critical appraisal phases: a) comprehension, b) content, c) variables & concepts, d) ethics.
2. Use four critical appraisal phases to evaluate single research studies.
3. Classify quantitative research evidence (experimental, quasi-experimental, non-experimental).
4. Use Critical Appraisal and Evidence Display Table Shells for data extraction.
5. Evaluate research [AACN essentials 4.1f].

Once article screening ends, researchers conduct a careful evaluation of each piece of evidence. The evaluation, called **critical appraisal**, is a complex, multidimensional process. The purpose for critical appraisal is to decide whether the evidence is credible, valid, and useful to answer the practice-based question. The fruit of competent critical appraisal is a clear, compelling evidence story. Wise researchers present two sides of the evidence story. They show the evidence that is present. They also point out what elements might be missing from the story.

This chapter covers four of seven major phases of the critical appraisal process for single research studies. Chapter 9 covers comprehension, content, variables and concepts, and ethics, with an emphasis on quantitative appraisal. Chapter 10 focuses on critical appraisal aspects such as methodology, analytics, interpretation of findings, and discussion, with an emphasis on qualitative appraisal. Each phase of critical appraisal has associated tasks. A summary of the basic critical appraisal process is shown in Appendix C.

Phase 1: Comprehension—First Reading

The first task of critical appraisal is comprehension. Researchers must read each article attentively and completely to know what each article says. First, arrange all articles in historical order, with the oldest articles first and the newest publications last. Once the articles are in order, researchers must take uninterrupted time to read each article completely. The full process of critical appraisal requires three separate layers of reading. Each layer of reading has a different purpose. Comprehension is the purpose of the first reading. The goal is to become familiar with everything in the body of evidence, including ideas that might not make sense at first. The first read is an immersion experience. Readers must learn the ideas, analytical strategies, strengths, and limitations of each article to know the entire body of evidence. Most importantly, they learn how each researcher interpreted and explained their own findings. A gift of the first full reading is that evidence-based researchers might find surprising subtopics within the evidence.

While reading each article for the first time, readers must ask critical questions. For example, does the article title match its content? Does the abstract match the content? Does the article contribute evidence to answer the PICO question? Is the article clear? Is the article confusing? Is it logically consistent? Does the article seem complete or are there any obvious missing pieces? An obvious missing piece would be if the researcher had four specific aims but only answered one. Three unanswered specific aims would be obvious missing pieces of that article. The idea of missing data related to social determinants of health are not obviously missing to the researcher. These are silences in the body of literature that need to be observed and noted. Once the silences related to social determinants of health are noted in systematic ways, they can be actively addressed.

This first reading gives researchers a chance to adjust their final evidence set. If researchers see that the article's title and abstract promised more than the article delivered, they might change their mind about that article's value. They might reject that article from the evidence set. Move such articles into a "not accepted" file. Do not delete "not accepted" articles. They might become valuable later.

Number all articles for the final evidence set with a two-digit format [01, 02, 03]. Enter article numbers in the top row of the evidence display table shell. Create the numbered references key with the same two-digit format to put beneath the evidence display table shell. The reason for a two-digit format is to avoid autocorrect complications if the number of articles exceeds the number 9. In some computers, going from the number 9 to 10 reorders the 10th, 11th, 12th items in second place after a single digit 1. The order will look like this: 1, 10, 11, 12, 2, 3, 4. Using a two-digit format preserves the number order of references. Once the table shell is set up, duplicate the basic evidence display table shell ten times.

Name each evidence display table and save as separate files. The categories of display tables are 1) Interventions; 2) Outcomes; 3) Benefits; 4) Adverse Events; 5) Human Costs; 6) Economic Costs; 7) Types of Evidence; 8) Social Determinants of Health; 9) Complete Evidence Summary; and 10) Final Synthesis.

Researchers need enough blank critical appraisal shells to equal the number of articles in the final body of evidence. Each critical appraisal table shell starts with the article number and complete article reference. Researchers create the final reference list using either American Psychology Association (APA) format or another accepted format. For APA format, list references in alphabetical order by author last name. At the end of the presentation to stakeholders, place the list of all references at the end of the PowerPoint presentation. Save one version of the reference list in APA format. Researchers who use a reference management system, such as RefWorks or Zotero, can generate reference lists quickly.

Phase 2: Content—Second Reading

Once all table shells have been created, researchers are ready to read each article in-depth. During the second reading, researchers extract data and enter it into tables. Complete the critical appraisal tables first. The example in Table 9.1 shows a critical appraisal of a descriptive research study by Italian researchers about the early weeks of COVID-19. Each element of the appraisal is explained after the table. Please take time to review the critical appraisal table. The details will help readers learn how to read articles for their own critical appraisal work.

Keep in mind, the first goal for each critical appraisal is to decide whether to retain or reject the article. That decision is made after the first full reading. It is based on whether the evidence is credible and useful. During Phase 2 researchers get to know the content of each article by completing a critical appraisal table (see the example in Table 9.1).

Phase 3: Variables and Content

A second goal of the critical appraisal process brings researchers to Phase 3, Concepts and Variables. In Phase 3, researchers extract bits of evidence from the articles, sort them into categories, complete the evidence display tables for each article, and finally, rate each article's quality. In Phase 3, creating the evidence display tables is a process of fragmenting the evidence, sorting it, and building it in new ways via separate tables.

TABLE 9.1. Critical Appraisal Example

01	Grasselli et al. (2020). Baseline characteristics and outcomes of 1591 patients infected with SARS-CoV-2 admitted to ICUs of the Lombardy region Italy. *JAMA Network*, 323(16), 1574–1581.				
Category of evidence Research Single non-experimental study Type 3 Method Quantitative Non-experimental, retrospective case analysis	Sample Population: Symptomatic COVID+ patients from 72 ICUs in Lombardy region Italy Feb 20–Mar 18, 2020 Sample size: N = 1,591 Type of sample Convenience. Patients age 14–91, median age 63; mostly males Setting: 72 ICUs of Lombardy Italy	Variables Concepts Gender: 82% male Age: 60% > 61 years old Comorbidities: Mode of Resp Support 88% mechanical vent 11% noninvasive O_2 PEEP level [14–16 median] FIO2 [60% ages < 63; 70% ages > 63] PaO_2 FIO2/PaO_2 ratio ECMO [5 pts] Prone positioning [240/875] ICU LOS Mortality vs discharge Interventions: None, non-experimental Outcomes: 26% mortality 16% discharge home 58% still in ICU after 4 weeks Themes: 9% of all COVID-infected people needed ICU care (1,591/17,713)	Data collection Daily collection via telephone Analysis Univariate descriptive data plus demographics Instruments or measures Real-time PCR test for COVID	Findings HTN and Cardiovascular disease were significant comorbidities. Age > 63 years was significant. Male gender 82% significant. Strengths 72 ICUs from one hospital system in Italy, includes Roma & surrounding Lombardy region. All COVID+ patients admitted to 72 ICUs were admitted to the analysis. Limits: No power analysis: 58% pts still in the ICU after 5 weeks; study was over at 4 weeks, so final mortality might have been higher	Other info Authors compared their data with data from Wuhan and USA (Washington State) Author Interpretation Their sample of 1,591 ICU pts differed from other cohorts since 99% required resp support; however, in the hospital system, people who needed noninvasive resp support could be discharged home, unlike non-Italian systems.
Author credentials: 20 MD authors and one MS-educated author. All authors took active roles in data collection, management, and analysis		Reviewer's comments: A non-experimental, exploratory, retrospective descriptive analysis of a large sample. Careful daily data collection, analysis, and reporting of the experience of all COVID+ patients admitted to ICUs in a large system in Italy. Medications and SDOH data were not collected. Gender and age were significant. Mortality = 26%, still in ICU = 58%, so only 16% survived to discharge within the 4-week study period			Quality of evidence High: Consistent & clear findings. Well described

Details of Critical Appraisal Explained

It takes time and effort to learn something as complex as critical appraisal skills. The process of critical appraisal involves a thorough consideration of credibility, value, and usefulness of a research article for a specific purpose. Table 9.1 asks reviewers to record details about the article. While reading an article for a second time, reviewers would evaluate the quality of those details. Each research method, such as quantitative, qualitative, and mixed, has its own corresponding rules. Experienced researchers know those rules. They can see gaps, flaws, or inconsistencies in a research study that beginners cannot see. Therefore, each element of the critical appraisal above is explained in detail below, so readers will learn basic ideas about critical appraisal.

The article number and full reference are put at the top of the table. Start by examining the title and abstract. The title mentions baseline characteristics of ICU patients with COVID. Readers might realize, from the title alone, that this article is not an experimental or a quasi-experimental study. If it were, the title would have a phrase like "The Effect of X on Y" or "A Randomized Controlled Trial of ..."

Experiments or randomized controlled trials have at least two groups of people. Experimental groups receive experimental treatments, also called interventions or manipulations. A control group does not receive experimental treatment. For experiments, researchers collect and compare data from the two groups. From this title and abstract, readers can see this is not an experimental study. This study is about data collection from one group of 1,591 COVID-positive people in 72 intensive care units in Italy. This type of study is a non-experimental, descriptive study.

Someone might wonder, if the study is non-experimental, does that mean it is a nonresearch article? The title says the article is about characteristics of people. The title and abstract show that this article has statistical analysis of data from a large group of people. The authors received institutional review board approval for this study. Those facts make it quantitative research. The type of quantitative research is a descriptive, non-experimental research study. Non-experimental quantitative research is not nonresearch.

From reading the abstract, readers know that this is a retrospective descriptive study of cases. In fact, the title and abstract match the article's content exactly.

In the first column of the critical appraisal table, researchers must determine the type of evidence. See Figures 9.1 and 9.2 below.

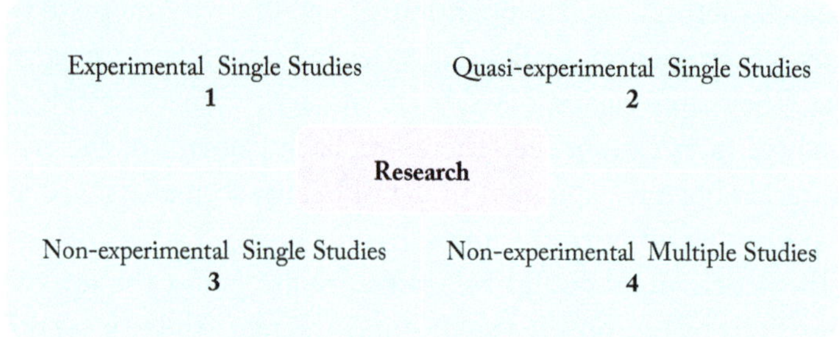

FIGURE 9.1 Categories of Research Evidence

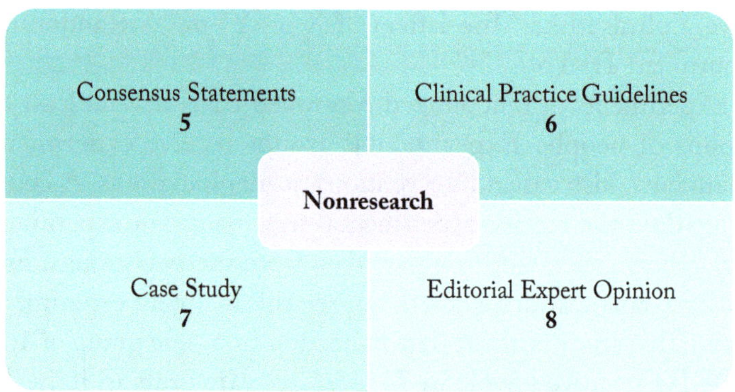

FIGURE 9.2 Categories of Nonresearch Evidence

The study is type 3, a non-experimental single study. The second column asks readers to describe four aspects of the sample: population, sample size, type of sample, and setting. Important questions for this category are as follows: Was the population of volunteers identified? In this case, yes. The sample is all severely ill COVID-positive patients from 72 intensive care units in a large hospital system in the Lombardy region of Italy. Was the sample described in sufficient detail? Again, the answer is yes. Demographic data, to the extent it was collected, is provided in the article. Elements of that data are further explained in the text. However, there is an issue about inclusiveness of data collection. It appears that the demographic data the researchers collected was completely reported. It also appears that there is hardly any information about most social determinants of health.

Does the sample represent the population? Yes, the authors addressed this issue. The authors recorded data on all COVID-positive patients in the large hospital system. No COVID-positive patients admitted to the ICUs were excluded. This was a total population, not a subset of the population.

Did researchers reduce sampling biases? In this case, yes. Was the sample size adequate for the study design and for the statistical analysis conducted? Yes. The sample size, N = 1,591, represented the total population for a 4-week period. This large sample permitted variability of human subjects. The statistical analysis was simple descriptive statistics, which is proper for a descriptive, non-experimental study. Was the sample size based on a power analysis? No. A power analysis was not needed since this was a simple, time-limited, retrospective descriptive study of the total population of patients in a large hospital system. A power analysis must be conducted when researchers plan to conduct certain statistical tests. Power analysis results tell researchers the ideal sample size needed to perform certain statistical tests with confidence. In this study, those kinds of statistical tests were not conducted. Rather, the data were analyzed for mean, median, mode, and quantities such as raw numbers and percentages. A power analysis was unnecessary.

In the third column, readers examine the article to find all relevant concepts, interventions, outcomes, adverse events. These aspects become the data bits that are extracted and put into separate display tables. Evidence display tables need the labels for each variable, and they need the "vote" to show that variable as present in each article that mentioned that variable. Variable labels go into the first wide column. Votes go in the vertical columns under the article number. Most researchers place an X to show which articles mentioned specific variables. Even though the Italian study did not have an experimental intervention, researchers collected data about patients' characteristics. The only demographic data were gender and age. Therefore, elements of demographic data missing from this study include employment status, marital/relationship status, home situation, family position (child, parent, sibling), social support, urban/suburban/rural geographic origin, racial/ethnic. These data categories that were not included might be mentioned on the social determinants of health (SDOH) display table as missing data (see Table 9.2 below). Medical information included comorbidities and specific respiratory assessment tests. The study did not include data about patients' smoking or vaping habits, alcohol consumption, or

TABLE 9.2 Evidence Display Table Showing Selected Elements Related to Social Determinants of Health That Are Missing from Consideration

Elements of SDOH	01	02	03	04	05
Employment status	0				
Food Security	0				
Housing Security	0				
Poverty	0				
Education level	0				
Relationship status	0				
Social support available	0				
Geographic origin	0				
Race/ethnicity	0				
Health care access	0				
Primary care access	0				
Health Literacy	0				

KEY: *01 Giacomo, 2020; 02 Author, year; 03 Author, year; 04 Author, year; 05 Author, year;*
NOTE: *X = information present; 0 = information missing*

use of nonprescribed drugs. The display table that shows patients' characteristics can also list data elements that might have been collected but were not.

The fourth column of the critical appraisal table addresses how data were collected and analyzed and whether the instruments or measures used were valid and reliable. Authors reported using a valid, reliable test for COVID-19. They reported a daily data collection process via telephone calls. Data collection via phone resulted in occasional missing data, but not a significant amount of missing data. The authors said that statisticians verified the data analysis. These factors increase confidence in the data shared in this article.

Findings are recorded in the fifth column. This study had strong, consistent findings. When evaluating statistical findings, results must be reported with all relevant data, such as the p value, which gives statistical significance for test results, or confidence intervals. In this case, there were no tests that could give a p value. However, the authors reported confidence intervals and raw numbers with percentages. The authors used easy-to-read tables with graphs to show findings. The tables, graphs, and text are consistent, strong, and clear.

To interpret their findings, authors compared their study data from Italy with data reported from Wuhan, China, and Washington State, U.S. The authors came to logical conclusions based on the data reported. In conclusion, this study is appraised as a high-quality descriptive, retrospective research study. The study has clear, consistent findings. The procedures, data collection, sample, and findings were all well-described. Finally, the authors compared their study findings with research reports from Wuhan, China, and Washington State, U.S. An evidence-based researcher who would use this article as evidence could have confidence in this article and its findings. Nevertheless, this article is missing the social determinants of health data. The inability for readers to know whether some of the people in this study were homeless or impoverished or had other factors impacting their health status is a lost opportunity.

Critical appraisal, as noted above, takes time and effort to learn. Eventually, critical appraisal becomes one of the most interesting aspects of evidence-based research. But in the beginning, as in this chapter, it might seem daunting.

Phase 4: Ethics

The Italian authors received institutional review board approval. Since data were collected passively and retrospectively, the review board approved data collection without informed consent. This element of ethics approval is essential to all reported research. For the above study, that element was met.

A different issue in the United States is related to our national effort to address social determinants of health and to increase diversity, equity, and inclusion in health care. An evidence display table for social determinants of health is included in Table 9.2. Most elements of social determinants of health are missing from the demographic data collected. As noted earlier, there is no mention of economic stability (employment status, income level), neighborhood and built environment (homelessness or urban, suburban, rural location of home), education access and quality (educational level), social and community context (relationship status, parental status, social support), or health care access and quality. These categories of social determinants of health are from the US Healthy People 2030 report (U.S. Department of Health and Human Services, n.d.). The research report was from Italy, not the United States. However, the social determinants of health ideas used in the United States are in sync with the social determinants of health advocated by the World Health Organization. The pressure for authors to collect and analyze key elements of medical data related to patients' respiratory needs is evident. Still, the lack of information in the report is a limitation of the study unrecognized by the authors.

Creating an evidence display table to show the social determinants of health elements that were missing from the study could provide evidence of another kind. Placing zeros to signify the lack of data could become a key indicator as more studies about early COVID are compiled.

After Critical Appraisal—Next Steps

After completing all critical appraisals, the next step is to complete the evidence display tables. The study above was descriptive, not experimental. It did not have any experimental interventions. Yet, an intervention evidence table can be completed for the study. In this case, interventions include all the variables for which data were collected. For example, mechanical ventilation, noninvasive respiratory treatments, and prone positioning are interventions, not outcomes. Another type of "intervention" was patients' baseline condition: comorbidities, age, and gender. To include elements such as comorbidities or demographic data, create a table called Patients' Baseline Conditions. Three outcomes for the study were 1) mortality, 2) discharged home, and 3) remained in the intensive care unit after the study ended. If there was a study 02, it might have the same or different interventions and outcomes. To complete display tables, researchers list all interventions in the first wide column of the display table. They would prepare the outcome display table in the same way. Then researchers would put an X in the article's column on any lines that match an intervention or outcome for that article.

Telling the Evidence Story

To tell an evidence story in a logical way, arrange the articles in historical order, with the oldest articles first and the newest articles last. This order helps researchers during appraisal and analysis to see how variables, theories, and ideas have evolved over time. When the final "evidence story" is presented to stakeholders, they will see how ideas evolved and where the evidence stands now. Presenting the evidence story in this way paves a logical path to final advice. If changes are advised, stakeholders will see the need more easily with a logically ordered evidence story than if the evidence story is randomly told.

Phase 3 Resumed: Data Extraction for Evidence Display Tables

Data extraction to build evidence display tables involves additional careful review after each critical appraisal. People have diverse ways of extracting and sorting different pieces of evidence. Evidence needed to answer or discuss the PICO question includes interventions, comparison interventions, and outcomes; themes found in the evidence; confounding variables; or novel ideas. Evidence tables show which articles contain specific elements of evidence.

Evidence display tables show the frequency and strength of elements found in the evidence. By looking at the tables, viewers could see whether variables increased, decreased, or changed, or if they cluster together.

The last and most important evidence table is the evidence synthesis table. Synthesis is a way to combine existing data in a new way. Analyze the display tables to understand the data deeply. Then put that new understanding in pictorial form in the final synthesis table. Pictorial form means to use specially created icons that give meaning to the data display. For example, use the colors of a stoplight: red for stop/negative, yellow for caution/no difference, and green for go/improved. Use symbols such as arrows up or arrows down. Use other small icon symbols to give meaning to the data on this table. Evidence synthesis forms the basis for any advice.

Once the evidence synthesis table is complete and advice is clear, make a final review of the evidence-based research project from beginning to end. This is when the third reading of the evidence occurs. With this final reading, having already extracted all relevant variables and outcomes, and having synthesized the data, the evidence-based researcher makes this last reading to make sure that the final advice given is well supported by the evidence.

Additional Points about Critical Appraisal of Individual Articles

If an article is research evidence, then the quality of research rigor will be important to assess. If the article is nonscientific, nonresearch scholarly evidence, then the credentials of the scholarly team involved in assembling that evidence are important, since there are no research criteria to assess. Articles obtained from library databases are considered external evidence since they originated outside of the researcher's organization. Internal evidence, which is evidence generated within a researcher's organization, is managed in a separate way.

The skill of critical appraisal of evidence, in any field, is difficult for most beginners to do. Appraising evidence is especially hard if someone has never produced any original research or nonresearch scholarly evidence of their own. Learning this skill depends on how well the person who appraises evidence understands the full process of how evidence is developed. However, the questions used to evaluate the research study above are important questions that must be asked of all types of evidence.

Research Rigor

When the phrase "research rigor" is used, readers might be prompted to focus on the word "rigor." They might think that studies with research rigor must have been hard to carry out or complicated or difficult. A rigorous study could be complicated or hard to conduct, but that is not what the phrase "research rigor" really means. Rigor refers to the precision with which a research study was conducted, whether it was a simple case study or a large, randomized controlled trial. Rigor has to do with thoroughness and excellence of the study, not with difficulty, obstacles, or complexity.

PURPOSEFUL PRACTICE EXERCISES

Learning Skill 4: Critical appraisal is not hard, but it takes practice, patience, and feedback. After reading this chapter, please engage in the **Purposeful Practice Exercises 9-1.** These exercises are set up to show what critical appraisal looks like and to practice this skill.

Summary

Chapter 9 presents in-depth details of how to conduct a critical appraisal, with emphasis on quantitative research. This book series uses an author-generated critical appraisal table shell and the Critical Appraisal Skills Programme (available at www.casp-uk.net). CASP tools are available online, free of charge. They are licensed under the Creative Commons Attribution: Noncommercial-ShareAlike. CASP tools include tools to critically appraise randomized controlled trials, systematic reviews, qualitative research, and cohort studies.

References

Grasselli, G., Zangrillo, A., Zanella, A., Antonelli, M., Cabrini, L., Castelli, A., Cereda, D., Coluccello, A., Foti, G., Fumagalli, R., Iotti, G., Latronico, N., Lorini, L., Merler, S., Natalini, G., Piatti, A., Ranieri, M. V., Scandroglio, A.M., Storti, E., … COVID-19 Lombardy ICU Network. (2020). Baseline characteristics and outcomes of 1591 patients infected with SARS-CoV-2 admitted to ICUs of the Lombardy region Italy. *JAMA Network, 323*(16), 1574–1581.

Hacker, K., Auerbach, J., Ikeda, R., Philip, C., & Houry, D. (2022). Social determinants of health—An Approach taken by the CDC. *Journal of Public Health Management and Practice, 28*(6), 589–594.

U.S. Department of Health and Human Services. (n.d.). Social determinants of health. Healthy People 2030. https://health.gov/healthypeople/priority-areas/social-determinants-health

CHAPTER 10

Skill 6

Critical Appraisal, Part II

LEARNING GOALS

1. Classify qualitative research as phenomenology, grounded theory, ethnography, or historical.
2. Critically appraise a qualitative research study.
3. Determine the quality of a research report.
4. Use critical appraisal results to rate the quality of research and nonresearch evidence.
5. Describe what interpretation of evidence means.

This chapter has five goals: First, explain four major categories of qualitative research. Second, demonstrate a critical appraisal of qualitative research that evaluates a narrative analysis style. Third, present criteria to determine the quality of a research report. Fourth, connect critical appraisal of narrative analysis to the skill of evaluating interpretive elements of research reports. Fifth, present individualized ways to determine the quality of research and nonresearch evidence based on current standards.

Researchers do not accept all research reports as valid just because they are published. Rather, researchers critically appraise each piece of evidence to determine its worth to answer a specific PICO question. The Critical Appraisal Skills Programme (CASP) began in 1993 in the United Kingdom. It is an open-access system with multiple critical appraisal tools online. CASP tools are set up with three sections of questions. The first question in section A of the CASP Qualitative Checklist is, are the results of the study valid? Section B asks, what are the results? Section C, will the results help locally? This last question is unexpected. The usual question for quantitative findings is, are results generalizable? This difference in that final question is one indicator of how different quantitative and qualitative research strategies and goals are.

Broad questions give clear purpose to critical appraisal. Yet, broad questions are not enough to learn how to engage in critical appraisal. Reviewers need detailed knowledge about research to evaluate research reports effectively. The question about what the results are can be hard to answer if reviewers do not know enough research language. For example, researchers report quantitative results in statistical language that a reviewer might not know. Likewise, reports of qualitative results might lack enough context and meaning. Lack of knowledge about research methods can be an obstacle to conducting an adequate critical appraisal. This chapter presents basic information about qualitative research. The CASP Qualitative Appraisal Tool is used as a basis for qualitative critical appraisal.

Four Qualitative Research Methods

Anyone who wants to conduct critical appraisals of qualitative research must learn about four basic qualitative methods. The first method, phenomenology, is usually an interview-based form of research. Phenomenology has sub-categories, such as descriptive, interpretive, hermeneutic, and existential.

Researchers who use phenomenology conduct interview-based studies of peoples' lived experiences of a phenomenon. Research titles that begin, "A Lived Experience of …" are phenomenological studies. If researchers use van Manen's ideas, they write about lived experiences in four realms: lived body (corporeality), lived space (spatiality), lived time (temporality), and lived human relation (relationality or communality) (van Manen, 1990). After interviewing people who have had similar lived experiences of a phenomenon, researchers transcribe and analyze the interview data. Qualitative researchers use a variety of narrative analysis strategies. If they use van Manen's ideas, they will analyze the interview data for elements of the lived body, lived space, lived time, and lived human relationship. When describing the results of their narrative analysis, phenomenologists discuss themes found in the data.

Due to the in-depth nature and length of qualitative interviews, phenomenological studies have small samples, about 10–12 participants. If a phenomenological study had few participants, for example only two or three, a reviewer would question whether there were enough data to draw conclusions. An ultra-small sample would make reviewers wonder whether the data and findings are skewed or biased. In-depth research interviews last on average about two or more hours. If a researcher reports interviews that lasted less than one hour, that would be a red flag that the interview was not in-depth. The reason that qualitative interviews can be so lengthy is that researchers often prepare a semi-structured interview. This means they plan a series of open-ended questions to answer the research question. Semi-structured interview questions must be substantial and probing. They must be open-ended. If interviewers ask questions that generate one-word responses, those questions are closed-ended, not open-ended. Two questions below show the difference (see Table 10.1).

With the closed-ended question, there are only two answers: yes or no. With the open-ended question, a respondent might give a short answer such as "Awful" or "Wonderful" or "Hard to say." An experienced qualitative researcher would encourage the person with

TABLE 10.1 Difference Between Open-Ended and Closed-Ended Questions.

Closed-ended	Did you graduate from high school?
Open-ended	Can you tell me what your experience of attending high school was like?

prompt questions such as "What do you mean?" or "Can you explain that in more detail?" There is nothing more for respondents to say after they have answered a closed-ended question. If researchers include the semi-structured interview questions in their research report, reviewers can see whether questions were open or closed.

A second qualitative method is grounded theory research. This method seeks to discover a basic social process. Grounded theory research involves procedures like constant comparative analysis of data, purposive or theoretical sampling strategies, data coding to break the narrative into smaller units, conceptualizing from the data, and developing a theory. A grounded theory research question starts with a broad, open question. As the study evolves, the question becomes focused. A typical sample size for a grounded theory study is about 25 people.

Grounded theory often uses interview-based data, but it can include other kinds of data, such as video data. Constant comparative analysis of data is a research strategy unique to grounded theory research. This means that after a researcher has interviewed the first respondent, the interview is transcribed and analyzed. After the first few cases, grounded theory researchers will know which characteristics the next participant should have. Purposive or theoretical sampling means the purposeful search for and enrollment of volunteers whose stories contribute conceptual elements to the theory. As each volunteer's data are collected, transcribed, and analyzed, researchers compare the data from interview to interview (constant comparative analysis). They seek participants based on ideas the researcher still needs to explore.

For example, if a researcher wants to conduct a study of women widowed 6 or more months ago, the researcher might enroll three women in their 80s widowed after their husbands suffered heart attacks or strokes. After the researcher has analyzed three interviews about women whose husbands died suddenly, the researcher might change directions. The researcher might wonder if widowhood is different for women whose husbands had a long terminal illness. The researcher might seek widows whose husband died 6 or more months ago after an illness of 3 or more years. That change in direction is why qualitative studies have emergent or flexible designs.

Qualitative researchers ask questions that are quite different from quantitative questions. Qualitative researchers do not interview a large random sample of people. They seek people who have specific life experiences to answer the research question. Qualitative researchers want to understand the full scope of knowledge for their question. Qualitative findings are not generalizable to populations. However, qualitative findings often inform researchers in ways that statistics are not able to do. For these reasons, qualitative researchers cannot predict the number of human subjects they will need. Rather, when they reach a point in their study called data saturation, they can safely stop enrolling volunteers. Data saturation means that the researchers no longer hear anything new in their data.

A third qualitative method is ethnography. Ethnographic researchers enter a culture or a community as outsiders, to become participant observers. Ethnographies are usually longitudinal studies. As participant observers, researchers enter with the outsider's point of view, also called the etic perspective. They collaborate with key informants to learn about that culture or community. During the study, ethnographers typically keep logs, take field notes, and write reflective notes at the end of each day. As the research continues, researchers might realize they have "gone native." That phrase means the researcher has adopted the emic perspective, or the insider's point of view. "Going native" usually signifies the study's end.

A fourth qualitative method is historical research. Researchers use archives to access and analyze letters, personal items, or documents of historical value. Researchers interpret the historical aspect through the artifacts they examine.

Over time, each of the four methods has evolved. The periodic reinterpretation of methods produces new variations. Critical appraisal of qualitative research takes time and effort to learn. The adequacy of critical appraisal is in how well reviewers understand the details of different research methods. It is important to know how quantitative and qualitative methods differ from each other. Grasping that difference is important for proper appraisal of research reports (see Table 10.2 below).

TABLE 10.2 Differences Between Quantitative and Qualitative Research

Quantitative Research	Qualitative Research
Uses a fixed or structured design. Changes to the design must be approved by the IRB.	Uses an emergent design that evolves while the study is underway.
Uses experimental, quasi-experimental, or survey methods to collect numeric data.	Uses interviews or participant observation to collect narrative data.
Collects numerical data for statistical analysis.	Collects interview data for narrative analysis.
Samples are large, random, anonymous if possible, with a firm number of volunteers needed.	Samples are small, handpicked, with an unclear number of volunteers needed.
Sample size is determined with a power analysis based on the planned statistical tests.	Sample size is determined when researchers believe they have reached data saturation.
Establish the statistical analysis plan before the study begins.	The narrative analysis plan involves multiple layers.
When planning the study, researchers anticipate and control to prevent confounding variables from affecting the data.	When conducting the study, researchers look for consistency and contradictions within interview data to decide on confirmability.

Critical Appraisal of a Qualitative Research Study

Critical appraisal depends on reviewers who know basic ideas about distinct types of research. Qualitative research, as noted above, is unlike quantitative research. A main difference between qualitative and quantitative research is the kind of design each type has. Quantitative research uses a highly structured plan to collect numerical data. Qualitative research uses an emergent design (also known as a flexible design) to collect narrative data. That means that qualitative researchers take each next step in a study based on information from earlier steps. The process of qualitative research often has a back-and-forth pattern. Qualitative researchers enroll volunteers and collect data until they have reached a point called data saturation. When researchers are no longer hearing any additional information, they stop enrolling volunteers. For the critical appraisal of a qualitative study, the CASP Qualitative Appraisal Tool asks 10 questions with multiple sub-items that help novice reviewers conduct a balanced review. The critical appraisal table below (Table 10.3) was completed for a qualitative study published in 2023. In that study, three academic nurses interviewed a sample of people (N: 18) who survived COVID-19 after an intensive care unit admission between March and September 2020. Please refer to Table 10.3 during the discussion of the CASP Qualitative Appraisal Tool (not shown).

The CASP Qualitative Appraisal Tool has three sections. Section A asks, are the results valid? To answer this item, the tool gives six sub-questions with hints. The first item is whether there was a clear statement of the aims of the study. For example, did the authors mention the study goal? Did the authors explain why it was important to do this study? This is difficult to answer from the research report. The authors described much about the onset of the COVID-19 pandemic, but they never specified exactly what they wanted to find out from the patients they interviewed. The choices on the CASP tool are "Yes," "Can't Tell," and "No." I would have to select "Can't Tell." Next item: Is the qualitative methodology appropriate? For this, my answer is Yes. To understand patients' experiences, a narrative-based study with semi-structured interviews is an effective way to obtain such information. However, the researchers did not specify their qualitative method. Next item: Was the design appropriate to address study aims? Yes and No. The idea of interviewing people by telephone with a semi-structured interview is good. However, their interviews were shorter than a usual qualitative interview. Their interviews lasted 30–45 minutes. High-quality qualitative interviews last 2 hours or more.

TABLE 10.3 Critical Appraisal Example of a Qualitative Study

01	Kurtuncu, M., Kurt, A., & Arslan, N. (2023). The experiences of COVID-19 patients in Intensive Care Unit: A qualitative study. *OMEGA—Journal of Death and Dying*, 87(2), 504–518.				
Category of evidence Research Non-ex-perimental, Qualitative Method Qualitative, Exploratory unspecified method	Sample Population: COVID+ pa-tients who sur-vived ICU stays from March to September 2020 14 males 4 females Sample size: N = 18 Type of sample Purposive Setting: Hospital in Turkey	Variables Concepts Theme 1: Feelings re: Illness & ICU Fear of death (16 of 18) Refused to believe they had COVID Fear of being alone Theme 2: Psychological & Physical Damage Witnessed nakedness; felt as if going mad; physical decline post-discharge Theme 3: Nurses' Efforts Value of Nursing care Theme 4: Protecting Life & Health Happy to survive/be alive, but cautious in mingling, crowds Interventions: N/A Outcomes: N/A Themes: 1. Feelings about illness & intensive care 2. Psychological and physical damage 3. Nurses' efforts & importance of care 4. Protecting life & health	Data collection Semi-struc-tured telephone interviews, 30–45mins/in-terview Analysis Authors worked together to tran-scribe, analyze data; used Miles & Huberman's data display Instruments or measures: N/A	Findings Communication from nurses to patients was key element of patient experience worth emphasizing Strengths Patients & research-ers did not know each other previously Authors did an exten-sive literature review, pre/post interviews Limits: Semi-structured interviews were 30–45 minutes via telephone; 5 broad questions	Other info Received ethics committee approval Octo-ber 2020, and informed vol-unteers about the nature of the study Author Interpretation Authors believed they might have had better interviews in a face-to-face manner. .
Author credentials: Three nursing faculty, Turkey, worked in triangulated manner to conduct this study.		Reviewer's comments: This was an exploratory qualitative study, with an unspecified method. Researchers used telephone interviews with five broad questions. Themes and questions are highly related. This calls into question the depth of interviews and of the analysis.			Quality of evidence Low–medium

The appraisal next asks if the recruitment strategy was appropriate. Yes. The authors reported a clear process for recruitment and enrollment with inclusion and exclusion criteria. Next item asks if data collection addressed the research issue. The report is unclear. Authors explained the limitation of using telephone interviews since face-to-face was not possible. However, their interviews were short, about 30–45 minutes, with five questions. The authors did not have any prior relationship with the volunteers, which reduces bias.

Section B of the CASP Qualitative Appraisal Tool has the overarching question of, what are the results? The sub-questions in this section focus on ethics, rigor of data analysis, and a clear statement of findings. The authors met the ethical concerns and rigor for data analysis very well. The authors describe a multilayer, triangulated data analysis strategy. Each author separately analyzed all interview data. Three authors discussed their data matrices. Authors collaborated throughout the data analysis to resolve any discrepancies. Three researchers used rigorous data analysis strategies. However, the depth of the interviews is an underlying concern. The findings reported were clear.

The last section of the CASP Qualitative Appraisal Tool asks about the value of the research. To understand the value of a qualitative study, reviewers must consider the quality of the discussion section of the research report and the conclusion. In this matter, the three authors wrote a robust discussion of their findings. The authors' conclusions related to the quality of communication during a time of isolation and alluded to the role that nurses played during the absence of visitors. Overall, the study has merit, with one lingering concern about the depth of the interviews.

Quality of a Research Report

One reason to conduct a critical appraisal of any evidence is to determine whether that evidence is credible and useful to answer a specific PICO question. How would a reviewer know objectively that a research report is credible? What criteria could a reviewer use to determine the quality, and therefore, the value of each piece of evidence?

During critical appraisal, readers ask themselves questions about aspects of each piece of evidence. Is the research report clear and convincing? Does the report tell a logical story, or are there contradictions within the story? Is the research strong, with substantial evidence to support clear findings? Is the research weak or flawed? Do the findings lack sufficient support?

Each piece of evidence must be evaluated according to the type of evidence it is. Research evidence is appraised according to the expectations of the type of research study. Nonresearch evidence is appraised according to the type of scholarship. Research, as noted above, can be separated into quantitative and qualitative categories. Each research category is based on opposite philosophical ideas. The underlying basis for the type of study could be a fixed, highly structured, quantitative study. Or the underlying basis could be an emergent, flexible, unstructured qualitative study. Reviewers must evaluate the strength of the research question and how well the study was designed to answer that question. Reviewers look at how volunteers were recruited and enrolled to see if study procedures were appropriate to data collection. Reviewers examine the approach to data collection, management, and analysis. With quantitative studies, reviewers would examine the statistical plan. With qualitative studies, reviewers would notice the layers of narrative analysis. Results are an important indicator of whether the study question was answered in a clear, credible way. More importantly, researchers' interpretations of their study's results and their mention of the strengths and limitations of their study are key features to determine credibility of the findings. After researchers have concluded a study, they are the ones with an inside understanding about things that were great and things that could have been better during the conduct of their study. Occasionally, researchers seem unaware of their study's limitations that reviewers can see so easily.

What Is Interpretation?

Interpretation is an analytical skill that sees beyond mere statistics or narrative themes. Interpretation gives meaning to statistics or themes. Lindgren and collegues (2020) wrote that "Interpretation can be defined as a process that involves explaining, reframing, making sense of, or otherwise showing an understanding of ..." (p. 2). That is a perfect description of interpretation.

Explaining study results requires basic knowledge about either statistics or narrative analysis. Consider a researcher who conducts an experimental study. Before the study begins, the statistician advises the researcher that at least 350 people will be needed for each group to obtain a credible statistical result with significance. If the researcher enrolls only 35 people for each group and collects data, how will that small sample affect the results?

With such a small sample, a researcher would not be able to conduct the original statistical tests. The researcher could use an alternative statistical plan. The alternative plan might make it difficult to fully answer the original research question. But what if the researcher was able to enroll 325 people in each group? That is close to 350 in each group. Is that sample size good enough? No. The power analysis gave the least number that must be enrolled, so a sample of 325 in each group is too small for the results to be reliable, valid, and meaningful.

If research study results seem highly credible but the p value indicates no significance, what meaning would authors give to those final findings? They would interpret the final findings as not significant, especially if their sample size were adequate.

When considering the significance of results, is the p value the only thing? No. The p value is one indicator of statistical significance, but it is not an indicator of the clinical significance of the findings. Significance of findings depends on what the findings mean. Likewise, for qualitative studies, are all final themes significant? Again, it is important to know what the theme means in terms of the original research question.

References

Critical Appraisal Skills Programme (2018). CASP (Qualitative Critical Appraisal) Checklist. [online] https://casp-uk.net/checklists/casp-qualitative-studies-checklist-fillable.pdf.

Kurtuncu, M., Kurt, A., Arslan, N. (2023). The experiences of COVID-19 patients in Intensive Care Unit: A Qualitative Study. *OMEGA—Journal of Death and Dying*, 87(2): 504-518.

Lindgren, B.-M., Lundman, B., & Granaheim, U. H. (2020). Abstraction and interpretation during the qualitative content analysis process. *International Journal of Nursing Studies, 108*, 1–6.

van Manen, M. (1990). *Researching Lived Experience: Human Science for an Action Sensitive Pedagogy*. State University of New York.

CHAPTER 11

Skill 7

Synthesize Evidence

LEARNING GOALS

1. Explain what synthesis is.
2. Identify the elements of evidence-based research that foster synthesis skills.
3. Grasp the meaning-making role that synthesis brings to evidence-based research.
4. Develop evidence synthesis tables.
5. Use synthesis skills to write the end of the evidence story.
6. Interpret evidence findings.

What Is Synthesis?

Synthesis means to combine two separate things to make a new thing. For example, when chemists combine two types of chemicals, they can make a synthetic material called polyester. Chemically based synthetic fabrics were invented during the 20th century. Today, clothing manufacturers use polyester, a synthetic fabric, to make clothing. Tire companies use polyester fibers to manufacture car tires. Synthetic materials like polyester have multiple uses.

However, polyester fibers do not occur in nature. Fibers that occur in nature are wool and cotton. Synthetic materials are fabricated (synthesized) in laboratories from chemicals.

When two ideas are combined (synthesized) into a new idea, scholars create new insights. For example, consider the idea of bed-sores. For more than 160 years, bed-sores have been attributed to inadequate nursing care of bedridden people. Nightingale wrote:

> If a patient is cold, if a patient is feverish, if a patient is faint, if he [sic] is sick after taking food, if he has a bed-sore, it is generally not the fault of the disease, but of the nursing care. (1859, p. 6)

Immobile, bedridden people can develop wounds. Two common names for those wounds during the 19th and 20th centuries were bedsores and decubitus ulcers. A variety of strategies to treat bedsores existed. Treatments were tied to what people thought caused bedsores. Previously, people thought bedsores were a result of patients lying too long in urine-soaked sheets. The idea was that when acids from urine contacted people's skin, sores developed. When antacids were developed, some nurses painted antacids on the people's wounds to neutralize the acids. Another thought was that moisture from urine would damage skin. With that idea, some nurses used lamps with hot electric lights to dry out wounds.

The bedsore/decubitus ulcer problem was unsolved until the late 1980s. A nurse, Barbara Braden, who cared for frail patients in long-term care settings studied this problem. Braden studied six factors, such as immobility, incontinence, skin turgor, and more. Braden collaborated with another nurse, Nancy Bergstrom. They developed the Braden Scale to detect risk for pressure ulcers, published in 1987. Braden and Bergstrom's work changed how nurses thought about bedsores. Things changed quickly after that. Nurses stopped talking about bedsores or decubitus ulcers. Nurses began using the phrase "pressure ulcers."

By looking at all the possible risk factors, Braden took apart all the ideas and concepts. When she synthesized the data in a new way, Braden had a new idea about patients' skin tissue tolerance.

That new idea helped people understand that if someone's skin were ultra-frail, it could not tolerate pressure like someone else with skin that was strong, especially in the setting of those six risk factors (Bergstrom et al., 1987). Nurses began preventing pressure ulcers in a new way. Using the Braden Scale to assess patients' risks for developing pressure ulcers, nurses took clear actions to prevent pressure ulcers.

The change in language spread beyond nurses. Hospital bed companies stopped using hard mattresses packed with horsehair and covered in heavy vinyl. Hospital beds and mattresses were redesigned to reduce pressure. By combining the idea about frail patients' tissue tolerance with the idea about pressure from hard mattresses, Braden and Bergstrom's synthesis of ideas and their insight about tissue tolerance changed how nurses worked and which mattresses were bought and sold. This example shows how synthesis (combining ideas in a new way) works.

Elements of Evidence-Based Research That Foster Synthesis

After critical appraisals are complete, researchers should know the big and small ideas present in the evidence. They might be aware of missing ideas. The detailed setup of separate evidence display tables gives researchers a unique grasp of the evidence and its gaps. This is when evidence-based researchers check the logic of their evidence story for its beginning, middle, and end.

The multilayered work of evidence analysis takes researchers to the threshold of synthesis. Think about that. Chapter 5 explains how to write precise PICO questions and find close cousin words. That chapter helps readers decide whether terms are subjects, objects, or action words in a PICO question. Chapter 5's content supports synthesis because researchers immerse themselves in the concepts of their PICO question. Synthesis of ideas starts when researchers struggle to find the right words.

During database searches, researchers refine their own grasp of ideas when they develop inclusion and exclusion criteria. Remember how database searches are conducted in a back-and-forth way? Remember how researchers can take advantage of a database's unique features? Robust database searches give researchers the gift of keen understanding about relevant and irrelevant ideas. Remember the advice in Chapter 9 to read the evidence three times in three separate ways for three purposes? During critical appraisal, researchers create multiple evidence display tables. To do so, they take command of their evidence. They gather and sort pieces of evidence. Then researchers fragment the evidence to display it in separate tables. The process of critical appraisal and table development exposes researchers to expected and unexpected ideas. As researchers fragment and sort ideas to create separate evidence tables, they can have insights about how data might fit together in a new way. That is the evidence-based path to synthesis.

To understand the idea of fragmenting, sorting, and fitting the data together in a new way, consider how table shells are used. Display tables show where in the articles (and in time) the existing ideas occurred. This is why arranging articles in historical order, with the oldest publications first and newest last, is important. Display tables show the frequency of ideas across all the articles in the evidence set. How concepts cluster together in the tables is another clue about the evidence. For example, if there are five intervention tables but one outcomes table, that means that people are getting to the same ends from a variety of paths. By examining and sifting the data, researchers can see the value of certain ideas in the body of evidence. During synthesis, certain existing ideas become prominent. Through synthesis, those prominent ideas can lead to a new idea. The new idea has a meaning that each previous idea alone never had.

Grasp the Meaning-Making Role That Synthesis Brings to Evidence-Based Research

To make meaning from the data tables that have been assembled, researchers look for clusters of information. To create evidence tables, the evidence must be fragmented, sorted into categories, and sifted for any golden nuggets. Researchers cluster similar concepts and search for themes or patterns in the data. For example, when comparing two interventions, researchers might see the original outcome, such as an adverse event, with negative implications. That might prompt a researcher to wonder about a different, positive outcome. Creating a new context for the original PICO question is part of an analytical approach that leads to synthesis.

Patterns stand out on display tables as the frequency or density with which certain data elements appear. The pattern can lead researchers to rethink existing ideas. For example, when I conducted a qualitative study about moral distress (2001–2002), volunteers said their experience was "gut-wrenching." One volunteer said she felt "socked in the gut" (Hanna, 2002). That word, "gut," kept turning up in the data. It was a pattern. I began to wonder why people were mentioning their viscera. As I analyzed the data further, I saw those data as part of a larger pattern. First, people experienced the gut-wrenching feeling, the visceral sensation. Next, they experienced cognitive awareness, a sense of disbelief. My synthesis of these data led me to the new idea that the experience of moral distress starts with "visceral discernment." With visceral discernment, a person's body knew about their moral distress before their intellect knew (Hanna, 2005).

As I came to the end of the analysis, I considered those data from different angles. I looked for gaps in my own data. One afternoon, I thought that people who might have had exceptionally severe moral distress might have committed suicide. That means that people with extreme moral distress would not be in my study or anyone else's. That meant that I had studied survivors of moral distress. This was an insight into the data that I could not have planned. Yet, at the end of the study, when I knew more about the topic than I did at the beginning, that idea made sense.

During an evidence-based research project, researchers take command of the evidence. They spend time reading and re-reading the evidence. They pull data bits from the evidence to create multiple display tables. The process of fragmenting, sorting, and sifting data bits of evidence is key. Finally, they review the evidence story's logic from the evidence display tables. All the big and small ideas about that evidence are the context. That is when synthesis of evidence can occur. That is how evidence-based researchers formulate their most important table, the evidence synthesis table.

Creating Evidence Synthesis Tables

To create an evidence synthesis table, researchers start with a basic display table shell. After creating display tables for interventions, comparison interventions, patient characteristics, outcomes, and other factors, synthesis tables show what the evidence means. Like all other display tables, the data labels listed in the first wide column affect how people read the whole table. Synthesis tables use icons to show data contrasts for different patterns, themes, variables, interventions, and outcomes. Evidence display tables show how data cluster with various ideas. Evidence display tables set up in chronological order will also show whether any ideas are obsolete or have been overturned by current ideas.

If evidence display tables give researchers a way to break up and sort the evidence into separate categories, synthesis tables are where the pieces are put together in a new way. The synthesis table is the logical link between the evidence and evidence-based advice that researchers give to stakeholders. The synthesis must be valid, logical, useful, and credible.

Evidence Interpretation

The second logical link between evidence and evidence-based advice is interpretation. During the synthesis process, researchers put ideas together in a new way. Interpretation is the evaluative aspect, the researcher's conclusions about what the evidence says. An important element of interpretation is whether the evidence is sufficient to answer the PICO question. Given the search for social determinants of health information, a novel layer of evidence-based research, an important interpretation of the evidence will regard the capacity of this evidence set to support recommendations to improve health equity.

Ultimately, a researcher's interpretation of the evidence is an informed conclusion. Interpretation is not the same as unreasonable assertions. Interpretation may not go beyond the data examined. A researcher's conclusions must be consistent with and supported by the evidence.

Summary: Synthesis as a Basic Research Skill

To present evidence-based advice to stakeholders, researchers take apart and then rebuild all the variables, categories, and synthesized evidence into an easy-to-grasp story. When learning how to engage in critical appraisal, it is best to work in three stages. The first stage is comprehension, to understand the evidence story. The second stage is fragmenting, sorting, and extracting data bits of evidence, to place them into separate tables. The last stage is to creatively combine and synthesize the data, which means to put data together in a new way.

References

Bergstrom, N., Braden, B. J., Laguzza, A., & Homan, V. (1987). The Braden Scale for Predicting Pressure Sore Risk. *Nursing Research 36 (4)*, 205–210.

Braden, B. J. (1988). *The relationship between serum cortisol and pressure sore formation among the elderly recently relocated to a nursing home* (Publication No. 8909621) [Doctoral dissertation, University of Texas at Austin]. ProQuest Dissertations and Theses Global.

Hanna, D. R. (2002). Moral distress redefined: The lived experience of moral distress of nurses who participated in legal, elective, surgically induced abortions. (Publication No. 3053658) [Doctoral dissertation, Boston College]. ProQuest Dissertation and Theses Global.

Hanna, D. R. (2005). The lived experience of moral distress of nurses who assisted with elective abortions. *Research and Theory for Nursing Practice: An International Journal. 19*(1), 95–124.

Nightingale, F. (1859). *Notes on nursing: What it is and what it is not.* Harrison, Bookseller to the Queen.

CHAPTER 12

Skill 8

Evidence-Based Advice and Advocacy

LEARNING GOALS

1. Explain advice and advocacy.
2. Read the evidence story for achievable actions.
3. Classify types of advice or advocacy.
4. Collaborate with stakeholders to develop an achievable action plan.

Evidence-Based Advice and Advocacy

Evidence synthesis often guides researchers toward clear advice about best practices. No matter how clear the ideas are, advice is not a one-way deal. Evidence-based researchers have a duty to present the evidence story in a clear, unbiased, logical way. That gives stakeholders a chance to collaborate with researchers to develop an achievable action plan.

In the beginning of an evidence-based project, PICO questions focus on the pragmatic value of this work practice versus that work practice to achieve an outcome. The focus is distinctly narrow for a good reason. However, critical appraisal of the evidence for a specific PICO question could reveal large elements that were previously hidden from view. Stakeholders expect evidence findings to prompt immediate workplace actions. Yet, the evidence can reveal larger needs for advocacy beyond one's work environment. As evidence-based researchers start to include evidence display tables for social determinants of health, that larger context for change will appear. The larger context is where advocacy for social action and political engagement is visible.

Evidence-based advice for immediate actions must be feasible, logical, practical, clear, and achievable. Feasible advice is achievable, especially if resources for change are available. Yet, a question remains: If the evidence shows a need for changes in work practices, how much change is needed? Is the change a minor adjustment to work procedures? Minor changes can be quickly achieved. Or does the evidence point to larger issues? Is the advice at the level of organizational change? Large organizational changes require specific implementation projects. Is it even larger, at the level of societal change? Broad social change, which is both internal and external to an organization, requires advocacy and a plan.

Logical advice flows from evidence synthesis to specific actions. Such advice is often practical and clear. If the evidence story were well told, stakeholders would expect this advice. Besides being logical, changes that flow from the evidence story are more easily supported by others if the evidence is strong. John Kotter, professor emeritus at Harvard's School of Business, tells leaders to "create a sense of urgency" when work changes are needed (2008, p. 10). This means giving others a compelling reason to change.

Reviewing the Evidence Story for Achievable Actions

When reviewing the evidence story for achievable actions, it is important to know which categories of actions exist. For PICO questions derived from clinical or client situations, the achievable actions could be work practice changes, either of processes, policies, or both. Besides changing direct work practices, additional advice could be related to providing more information or professional worker education to improve knowledge and, therefore, to improve professional performance. Advice might address improving communication strategies or supervisory practices. If the advice is to use new procedures, technology, communication strategies, or supervisory practices, a parallel piece of advice might be to retire current procedures, technology, communication strategies, or supervisory practices. If the PICO question was aimed at how professionals serve their clients, or if the PICO question focused on a comparison of two alternative interventions for clients, the variety of actions advised might include how to inform clients about their alternatives, how to help clients choose the preferred interventions, and how to evaluate the quality of service provided after advised interventions are implemented.

Researchers who examined their evidence for social determinants of health (SDOH) might advocate for ways to address larger issues that were previously hidden from view. Researchers who use the *Future of Nursing* SDOH model by Castrucci and Auerbach might advocate for changes in five categories of social determinants (Hacker et al., 2021, p. 37). They might also use three realms (upstream, midstream, and downstream) to better define the type of advocacy needed (see Table 12.1 below).

TABLE 12.1 Social Determinants of Health Categories and Specific Factors

Future of Nursing 2020–2030 Framework	
Categories	**Specific Factors**
Economic Stability	employment; food insecurity; housing instability; poverty
Education	early childhood education & development; enrollment in higher education; high school graduation; language & literacy
Social & Community Context	civic participation; discrimination; incarceration
Health & Health Care	access to health care; access to primary care; health literacy
Neighborhood & Built Environment	access to foods that support healthy eating; crime & violence; environmental conditions; quality of housing

The Future of Nursing model of SDOH shows researchers a three-pronged way to use evidence-based findings. Upstream strategies have a community impact. These strategies would be "improving community conditions and addressing adverse social determinants of health," (National Academies of Sciences, Engineering, and Medicine, 2021, p. 37). If an evidence-based study reveals the need for upstream strategies, Castrucci and Auerbach's theory recommends using "laws, policies and regulations" to "support health for all people" (National Academies of Sciences, Engineering, and Medicine, 2021, p. 37). Advocacy for upstream changes would occur both within and outside the organization.

Midstream strategies have an individual impact. These are strategies to address people's social needs. For nurses, social workers, and other health professionals, screening clients for factors like housing or food access might give professionals a chance to help individual clients in meaningful ways. Advice for midstream issues might be actions that straddle a health care organization and the surrounding community. Downstream factors occur inside the health care system after people have chronic or acute illnesses. At that point, people need direct medical and health care interventions. Therefore, downstream SDOH changes would occur within a health care organization.

Classify Types of Advice or Advocacy

For simple evidence-based research projects, work practices change in three ways. When a work procedure changes, organizations might require a new written procedure to reflect the change. A change in procedure might prompt a change in the policy that governs that procedure. If there is an underlying standard to support the procedure, this too might need to be rewritten. All three elements, the written procedure, policy, and standard will need approval at either an organizational or administrative level. Once the changes are approved, the next action would be to communicate the change to others who need to know that information. Also, if a new procedure is put in place, current procedures will be retired. If a new assessment or a new form of data collection is instituted as part of the achievable advice, and if current assessments or data collection procedures are retired, this requires approval and must be communicated to relevant work groups. If the change of procedure, assessment, or data collection affects organizational informatics or technology, then researchers must work with the information technology or organizational assessment departments to achieve those changes.

As advice for achievable actions is accepted, a crucial element of making change is paying attention to how such changes are communicated to relevant others. Organizations that anticipate change on a regular basis also provide ways to ensure that employees are aware of changes. Staff education might be an achievable action. Finally, it is important to plan for staff performance evaluation. This will help researchers and other stakeholders see whether the advice for change was accepted and used successfully.

From an organizational perspective, as changes are made to work practices, administrators might evaluate quality outcomes after the changes were implemented. Together with performance outcomes, they might evaluate cost efficiency, if any, and depending on the nature of the change, any new revenue generated due to the advised changes.

Collaborate to Develop an Achievable Action Plan

After presenting the evidence story, researchers might invite stakeholders to collaborate to develop an achievable action plan. The evidence-based research PowerPoint template is set up with three slides that show implications of the evidence. Not all listed implications will be relevant. The list is provided as a springboard for brainstorming and collaboration. Notice that the slides are titled Current Implications, Future Implications, and SDOH Implications. Current implications are the changes most immediately advised based on the evidence. Future implications refers to future effects if advised changes are made, and it includes possible other changes in the future that can be foreseen at the time of this presentation. SDOH implications are changes that must be considered, especially if the evidence uncovers previously hidden inequities.

Stakeholders and evidence-based researchers collaborate to finalize a plan for achievable actions. Once this plan is agreeable to all concerned, it is time to communicate the evidence story and the achievable actions plan.

References

Hacker, K., Auerbach, J., Ikeda, R., Philip, C., & Houry, D. (2022). Social Determinants of Health—An approach taken at CDC. *Journal of Public Health Management and Practice, 28*(6), 589–594.

Kotter, J. (2008). Sense of urgency: Incite inspired action. *Leadership Excellence, 25*(3), 10.

National Academies of Sciences, Engineering, and Medicine. (2021). *The future of nursing 2020–2030: Charting a path to achieve health equity.* The National Academies Press. https://doi.org/10/17226/25982

CHAPTER 13

Skill 9

Share Final Findings

LEARNING GOALS

1. Prepare professional presentation of evidence-based findings for internal stakeholders.
2. Prepare conference abstract for external professional presentation.
3. Communicate scholarly findings [AACN essentials 4.1g].

Once their projects end, evidence-based researchers must present their findings to the most immediate stakeholders. Those stakeholders are usually the researcher's direct work supervisor, who might have approved the researcher's time spent working on the evidence-based project, and work peers. If the evidence affirms current work practices, then organizational changes are not needed. Yet, the evidence-based researcher would still present their findings to work peers to confirm that current work practices are still advised. If compelling evidence shows that organizational change is advised, the evidence story will point toward specific ways to achieve such change.

Readers can use the PowerPoint template provided with this book as a basis for a public presentation of their study. The template is written to show the entire evidence story—beginning, middle, and end. Besides bringing closure to the original PICO question, presentation of evidence-based findings creates a friendly path to organizational change and work-based excellence.

When evidence-based findings show a clear need for organizational change, researchers must communicate those findings to all relevant stakeholders. This might mean making serial presentations to different departments or work groups, depending on the changes being advised. As researchers present final findings and advice to each stakeholder group, researchers should invite stakeholders to collaborate to develop the action plan to implement change.

Presentations of final findings that are logical, clear, and interesting can ignite a desire for change among organizational peers and stakeholders. According to Harvard professor John Kotter, the first effective step to organizational change is to "establish a sense of urgency" (2007, p. 99). In his follow-up 2008 article, "A Sense of Urgency: Incite Inspired Action," Kotter wrote, "You need more action from a broader range of people—action that is informed, committed, and inspired—to lead change." When evidence-based research is well executed, it is informed by strong, high-quality evidence. Robust evidence usually refers to a consistent pool of evidence that leads toward a unified answer. Presentations of such high-level findings can inspire others to take action together.

Readers must feel free to modify the PowerPoint template as needed. For example, if the evidence reveals a need to change work practices or work policies, researchers might emphasize that advice with a brief outline of how to change an existing practice or policy. It is possible that researchers might not realize who all the relevant stakeholders are until the project is complete. Evidence-based researchers might use their organizational chart to understand how different departments in the organization are connected to each other. This might help them see which departments to include in the presentations for all changes to be made.

For example, it might become clear at the end of a project that a purchasing agent might need current information to make a more informed purchase for the organization. Another example is that something that was formerly seen as a fluke of operations might finally be understood through new insights as an event to anticipate and prevent. One benefit of presenting the findings internally to all relevant stakeholders often comes as a surprise. When researchers invite everyone to join in developing the action plan and people feel welcome to contribute their ideas, achievable actions are more likely to become a welcome change.

Presenting Evidence-Based Findings Externally

Professional conferences are perfect venues to share evidence-based findings beyond one's immediate workplace. Two ways to present evidence-based findings at conferences are 1) with a brief podium PowerPoint presentation, and 2) with a poster presentation. Readers might need to trim the current PowerPoint presentation template to ensure that the presentation can be made in the allotted time. When preparing an abstract to present at a professional conference, follow the guidelines set by the conference organizers. Find out if your presentation will be in podium or poster format. It is possible to offer to present in either format at certain conferences, but if accepted, presenters are only afforded one presentation mode, not both.

For a podium presentation, the conference abstract guidelines will usually indicate the number of minutes for presentation and the number of minutes allocated for questions and discussion after each presentation. If the podium presentation is for either 5, 10, or 15 minutes, the PowerPoint slide presentation must have no more than one slide per minute. Also, each slide must be readable and useful. It is not useful to put every word of a 20-slide presentation onto five slides. Rather, it is possible to select the 5 or 10 or 15 most important slides to present in that given time frame. The rest of the slides can be hidden so that in the Slide Show format, hidden slides will remain intact within the presentation but will not be shown during the slide show. Hiding slides is a key element when giving a presentation, since keeping all the slides intact preserves the entire evidence-based research project. If anyone in the audience challenges a point that is on a hidden slide, it is possible to access that hidden slide immediately to show it to the audience member. Researchers are expected to complete an individual critical appraisal slide for each piece of evidence reviewed. However, during most presentations of final findings, researchers will show only one or two of the individual critical appraisal slides. The other critical appraisal slides are kept hidden during public presentations. However, if someone were asked to give their complete presentation for review (for example, to a direct supervisor), the entire PowerPoint with all slides intact could be shared.

The procedure to hide slides for a formal PowerPoint presentation is quite easy. Follow the screenshot images below.

Open the PowerPoint presentation. Go to the ribbon and click on **View**.

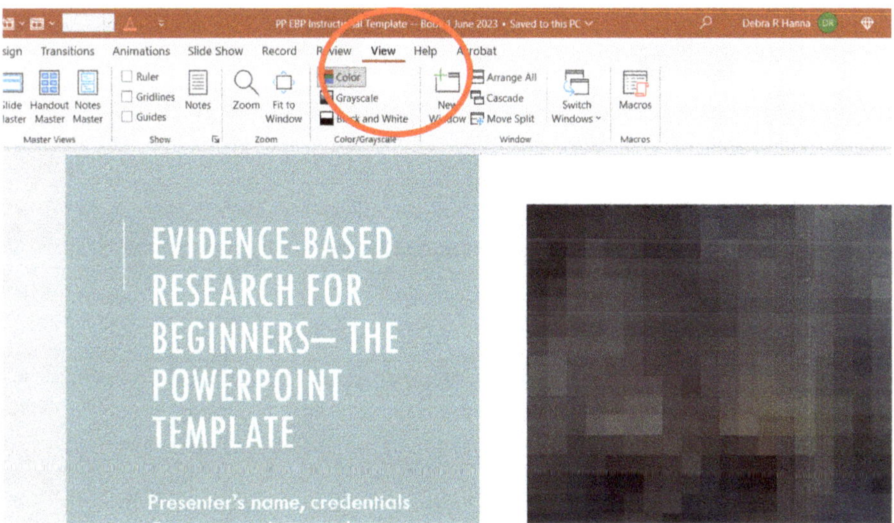

IMG 13.1

When the ribbon changes, click on **Slide Sorter**.

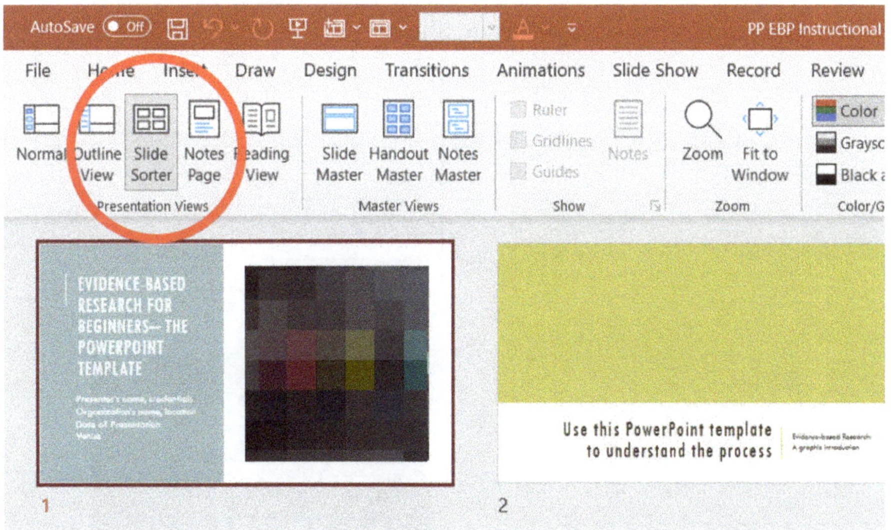

IMG 13.2

Scroll down to the slide to be hidden. Click on the slide while it is shown in the Slide Sorter format. A menu will appear. Click on **Hide Slide**.

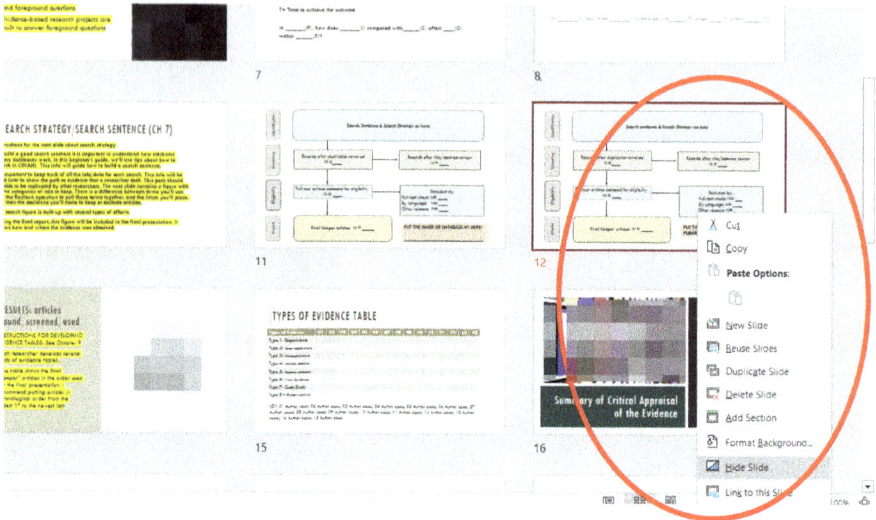

IMG 13.3

The slide number is crossed out to indicate that the slide is hidden from public view during a Slide Show.

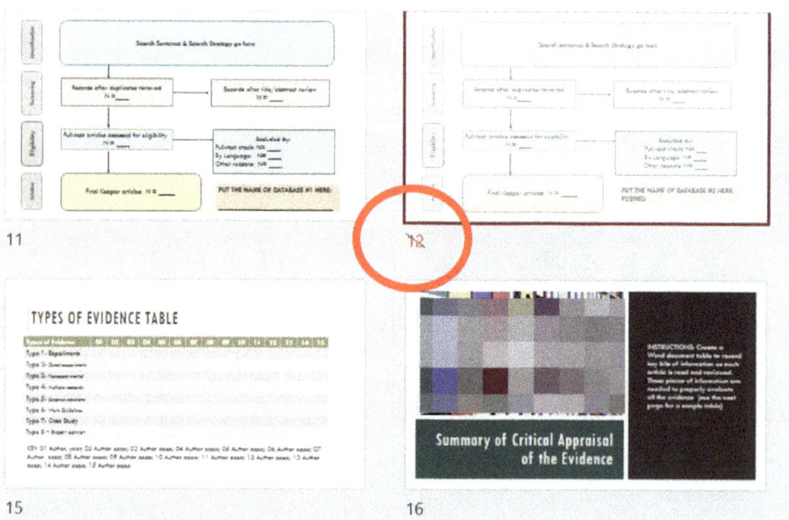

IMG 13.4

Finally, if the abstract is accepted for a poster presentation, the PowerPoint slides can be used to create a poster presentation. It is important to determine from the conference guidelines whether posters will be presented electronically or in a large-poster format in a hall. If the poster will be in electronic format, it is important to know whether the poster will be a single slide shown for less than 1 minute with other posters scrolling during the poster session, or if the poster will be a brief, multi-slide presentation for about 5–10 minutes. It is also important to find out if there will be an audio portion to the poster presentation or if the electronic poster will be silent. The electronic format and time permitted will give presenters an idea of what is possible to share in that format.

If posters are shown in a poster hall in person at a professional conference, it is important to find out the smallest and largest sizes allowed for the poster, if it will be appended to a standing poster wall, or if it will sit upright on a table. If the poster is appended to a standing wall, the size and weight of the poster must be considered when it is being designed. To attend foreign conferences with a poster, an ingenious method of transporting a poster conveniently during air travel is to have all the pieces of the poster designed in segments that are about 14 x 16 inches in size. These pieces can be secured in a large envelope and placed in either one's carry-on luggage or a large handbag. It is not advised to put the poster inside one's checked luggage, in case the luggage is temporarily misplaced.

This chapter described internal presentations of final findings to stakeholders and professional presentations in podium or poster formats. These are not the only ways to communicate final findings. Other ways to communicate final findings will be presented in book two and book three of this evidence-based practice series.

References

Kotter, J. P. (2007). Leading change: Why transformation efforts fail. *Harvard Business Review, 85*(1), 96–103.

Kotter, J. P. (2008). A sense of urgency: Incite inspired action. *Leadership Excellence, 25*(3), 10.

Credits

IMG 13.1–13.4: Generated with PowerPoint. Software is Copyright © by Microsoft.

PART III

Appendices

Blank Basic Evidence Display Table Shell

List the evidence category here	01	02	03	04	05	06	07	08	09

Key: *01 Author, xxxx; 02 Author, xxxx; 03 Author, xxxx; 04 Author, xxxx; 05 Author, xxxx; 06 Author, xxxx; 07 Author, xxxx; 08 Author, xxxx; 09 Author, xxxx.*

Basic display table shell. Each article in the definitive evidence set has a number at the top of each column, which corresponds with numbered brief references in the Key beneath the table. Only the first author's last name is placed in the key, to keep the key as simple as possible. The "et al." designation is not used.

To create an Evidence Display Table Shell: Create a table with 2 columns and 2 rows. Move the middle line slightly left to create a larger first column. Then move the right column toward the left to create a narrow column. Insert a new column to the right. Repeat right column insertions until there are enough columns to match the number of articles for the evidence table. On the top row, number the narrow columns in two-digit format 01, 02, 03 and so on. Insert enough rows beneath the bottom row to create the remaining table shell. Beneath the bottom row, create the key with the 2-digit article number and first author's last name for each article. Once the table shell is set up, this table shell can be copied for all the needed evidence display tables.

APPENDIX B

Blank Critical Appraisal Table Shell

<table>
<tr><td>01</td><td colspan="5">Author Name(s). (year). Article title. Journal Title, vol.# (issue #), page numbers.</td></tr>
<tr><td>Category & Level of evidence
Research 1, 2, 3, 4
Non-Research 5, 6, 7, 8</td><td>Method
Quant
Experimental
Quasi-experimental
Non-experimental
Qual
Phenomenology
Groundod Theory
Ethnography

Mixed Methods</td><td>Sample
Population

Sample size
N = ___

Type of sample</td><td>Variables
Concepts

Interventions (IV)

Outcomes (DV)

Themes</td><td>Data collection

Analysis

Instruments</td><td>Findings

Strengths

Limitations

Inter-pretation</td></tr>
<tr><td colspan="2">Author credentials</td><td colspan="3">Reviewer's comments:</td><td>Quality of evidence</td></tr>
</table>

The critical appraisal table is presented in Chapter 8. This table, created in Microsoft Word, can be easily replicated for critical appraisal of each individual piece of evidence.

APPENDIX C

Summary of the Critical Appraisal Process

Stage	Step	Dimension or task	Task with rationale
	0	Pre-appraisal task	Arrange all articles in chronological order, with the oldest first to newest last.
I	1	Comprehension	Read all articles once completely to understand what each one says. The first reading should be attentive and task free. Readers will become aware of the variety of ideas in the full set of articles.
	1a	EB project task after first full article reading	Determine whether each article is valuable to answer the PICO question. If yes, give the article a number. If not, set the article aside without a number. Put info for each accepted, numbered article into the main table shell and create a final reference list.
	1b	EB project task	Set aside each rejected article in a "discarded articles" file until the end of the project, when articles might be used in a separate way.
II	2	In-depth, focused reading with Data Extraction	Read each accepted article a second time with the intent to extract needed data. Do not combine in-depth reading and data extraction reading with the first reading. An evidence-based project can become unmanageable if researchers are unfamiliar with the body of evidence when creating tables.

Stage	Step	Dimension or task	Task with rationale
	2a	EB project task	Set up and duplicate the main display table shell at least 10 times. Rename the display table shells for different purposes. (See Table Shell section in Appendix A.)
	3	Ethical	Check each article for two major ethical dimensions: IRB approval and voluntary enrollment of human subjects with informed consent.
	3a	Ethical: SDOH	Check for presence or absence of social determinants of health data.
	4	Content, Concepts, Theories	Independent variables, dependent variables; confounding or extraneous variables; themes
	5	Methods	Quantitative: RCT, quasi-experimental; non-experimental Qualitative: phenomenology, grounded theory, ethnography, historical
	6	Analysis and Statistics	Statistical Tests & Assumptions Univariate descriptive Measures of dispersion Measures of central tendency Measures of shape Multivariate Correlation Difference
	7	Interpretation & discussion	Review strengths and limitations in the discussion section. Review the extent that the original research question was answered and that the specific aims were met.

Index

www.ingramcontent.com/pod-product-compliance
Ingram Content Group UK Ltd.
Pitfield, Milton Keynes, MK11 3LW, UK
UKHW021830270726
14058UKWH00001B/78

9 798823 308908